JN292110

Professional English in a Hospi
Essential English for Medical St

—— 必 携 ——
病院における実践
医療従事者のための基

著者 | **Marshall Smith**
佐藤伸雄

医療科学社

推薦のことば

　はじめに著者の紹介をさせていただきます。マーシャル・スミス博士は，保健科学大学で長年にわたり英語教授に携わってきました。その間，内外の保健学会でも積極的に学術活動を行ってまいりました。この経歴からみまして，彼が本書を執筆することは真に当を得ていると信じます。佐藤君と出会ったのは15年前の国際会議で，それ以来お互いに尊敬と友情を深めあっていることは私にとって喜びにたえません。彼はウィスコンシン大学病院附属の放射線技師学校で非常勤講師としての責務を果たし，私ども米国放射線技師教育者会議にも出席していますので，彼の名は私ども教育者の間ではよく知られています。本書の出版により彼の評価がさらに高まるものと信じます。

　本書は，医療従事者が患者さんに対して良きcaregiverとなるための案内役となることでしょう。文体は読んで面白く，内容は現実的でわかりやすい事例や用語に満ち，小テスト（quiz）や練習問題は内容の理解度を高めるのに役立ちます。また本書は，解剖や生理学，さらに診療画像・技術学の優れた必携テキストとなり，医療従事者に実践的で不可欠な知識を与える内容となっています。各章併せて病院環境で必要な医療をすべてカバーし，いかにそれに対処すべきかの答えを与えてくれます。特に圧巻は，救急医療の事例と筋骨格損傷の対処法です。国際会議の内容は会議参加者同士の交流に大いに役立つことでしょう。重要表現に指定された個所は完璧で，読者が現実に遭遇したときに大いに役立ちます。

　私は自信をもって皆様に本書を推薦いたします。医学関係の図書館にぜひ加えていただきたい1冊であります。学校においては本書を教科書として活用することにより，学生が多くの知識と情報を得ることと信じます。

Gregory L. Spicer, M.S., R.T. (R)
Manager of Radiology Training and Education
Clinical Manager of Nuclear Medicine, PET, and BMD
University of Wisconsin Hospitals and Clinics
Madison, Wisconsin, USA

自　　序

　本書は看護，医療衛生（技術）学部の学生，あるいは医療スタッフ（co-medicals）を対象として書かれたものであります。医学の進歩にともない，チーム医療が必須となり，その実施にあたっては，各専門職間に一貫した対応が必要となります。このためには，関係者が学際的な知識を共有し，意見や情報の交換を行い，個々の患者さんに最適な対応ができる体制づくりが必要です。これが実現されてこそ，専門職間のスムーズな協同作業ができるものと信じます。それには各専門分野に共通するテキストが必要となります。本書はこの観点から，とかく内向きな，あるいは特化した学問の垣根を取り除き，患者さんとの対話を通して英会話の力を養うとともに，教養課程の初期の段階から広い医療知識を身に付けることを目的としています。

　第1章の患者接遇と第2章の救急医療は，とかく本邦では学問として扱われがちですが，本書では，米国の医療系の学校で徹底して教えられている実用的な具体例を会話形式で紹介します。第3章は看護・栄養学，第4章は看護・臨床検査技術，第5章は放射線技術と理学・作業療法が中心となっていますが，全章とも他の専門職にも役立つ話題をとりあげています。第6章では，やがて訪れる病院の株式会社化，専門職の免許更新制度など，ホットな話題をディベート形式で紹介します。第7章は，先進国のなかで最も遅れている禁煙対策と，医療情報（会計情報，臨床検査や画像情報など）の統合化とペーパーレス・フィルムレスを目指した電脳病院の実現化に向けた話題を国際会議の討論でとりあげています。

　各章はリード文に始まり，その内容に関連する対話が続きます。対話に続き，小テスト（Quiz）が設けられています。これは，review questionであると同時に，患者さんとの対話形式では専門的すぎる内容を補足したものです。読者が質問と解答を反復朗読して英語によるQ&Aの自習ができるように，解答は設問の真下に置きました。章末のExerciseは文章問題で，各自が解答を作成するものですが，参考として模範解答を巻末に置きました。対話はできるだけ一般用語を用いましたが，対応する専門用語を（　　）のなかに，［　　］のなかには会話よりも解説的な専門的表現を入れました。各対話の後に続く"関連・補足表現"は，内容に関連する重要表現や慣用表現であります。特に患者さんや，外国の同僚との会話に欠かせない重要表現集を"付録"として別途に巻末に網羅しました。

　刊行にあたり，前例のない"ボーダーレス基本医療"を英会話テキストとして出版することにご同意くださった医療科学者の古屋敷信一社長，編集に尽力された齋藤聖之氏に深く感謝いたします。

　最後に，この書の刊行を見ることなくご逝去された北里大学の桜井清子教授にこの書を捧げ，ご冥福をお祈りします。

　　　　　　　　　　　　　　　　　　　　　　　平成15年秋　　　　著者記す

本書の使い方

> 本書は広範囲な専門領域を含んでいますので，特定の専門分野からみれば理解しにくい章があるようにみえます。そこで，下記のような利用法を提案させていただきます。

1. 教科書または副読本として利用される場合には，初めの2章は医療人としてどの分野にも必要な箇所となります。学年度の授業時間からみますと，残りのうち1章が自身の専門に関する章となります。その他の章は他分野の専門領域を垣根越しに覗く程度の気安さで時間の許すかぎりで消化されればよいでしょう。
2. 他分野の章については専門家を招待して講演してもらうのも良い方法かと思います。多くの看護師が海外留学されています。また，理学・作業療法士は指導者の多くが留学経験者で，放射線技師も留学経験者が増えてきました。教育の相互乗り入れで，本書が有効なチーム医療の礎となることを期待しています。
3. Quizは，本来は小テストという意味ですが，本書ではClause Reviewとして各項目（話題）ごとの内容をこの場で再確認するもので，やや高度な質問になっています。無理に回答する必要はありません。わからないときは，下に書かれている解答を読み上げることをお勧めします。そのときは，読んだ箇所が本文のどこに書かれているかを探して，その箇所をもう一度読み上げてください。あまり解答に時間を割くと授業になりません。内容は二の次にして，英語での質疑応答の形式を覚えることと，本文の重要部分にさかのぼる"手がかり"としてQuizを設けました。

略語と字体

i.e.：すなわち，言い換えれば

e.g.：例えば

cf.：参照，あるいは比較せよ

＊（注釈）：主にリード文中の専門用語の肩付きとして番号とともに付記

＠（特記，または蛇足）：注釈の域を超えた補足説明で，ときには意外さに＠（アッと）驚く説明でもある。

ボールド：専門用語にボールド（太字）を用い，＊ナンバーを肩付きにして和訳と対照させた。また部分和訳のなかで強調したい箇所をボールドで表示し，その箇所を拾い読みするだけでそのフレーズの概要が把握できるようにした（上記参照）。

イタリック：前記以外の特殊表現をイタリック体で表した。

INDEX 目次

推薦のことば
自　　序
本書の使い方
目　　次

Chapter I. Interaction with patients ········· 1
患者接遇法

1. Building mutual reliance ········· 1
──信頼関係の構築

Dialogue ········· 2

Relevant expressions and additional phrases ········· 6

1) Subjunctive Mood　仮定法

2) Causative Verbs　使役動詞

3) Collective Nouns　集合名詞

4) Expressions for mutual reliance　信頼関係に関する表現

5) Expressions for a cautious attitude　慎重な態度に関する表現

6) Taking accountability　説明責任を果たす

2. Interacting with children and elderly patients ········· 8
──子供と老齢患者への対応

Dialogue ········· 9

Relevant expressions and additional phrases ········· 11

1) Expressions of behavior　態度に関する表現

2) Understanding patient's physical and mental conditions
患者の様態・気持ちを察する

3) Psychological and physical aspects of eye level
心理的な目線と物理的な目線

4) Difference between Watch and See　WatchとSeeの違い

5) A state of mental incapacitation　のぼせの状態

3. Dealing with a terminally ill patient ········· 13
──末期患者への対応

    Dialogue ········· 14

    Relevant expressions and additional phrases ········· 18

        1) **Expressions of anger**　怒りの表現

        2) **Psychological leading**　心理的誘導

        3) **Flat and involved attitudes**
           素っ気ない態度と深入りしすぎた態度

        4) **Passing time**　時間的経過

4. Stress management ──ストレス管理 ········· 19

    Dialogue ········· 20

    Relevant expressions and additional phrases ········· 23

        1) **Cause and effect**　原因と結果

        2) **Link words**　つなぎ言葉

        3) **Emphasis by interrogative and negation**
           疑問・否定による強調表現

        4) **Singular or plural**　単数か複数か

        5) **Indefinite pronoun**　不定代名詞

        6) **Plural objects**　複数対象

Chapter II.　Emergency ········· 25
        救急医療

1. First Aid ──応急手当 ········· 25

    Dialogue ········· 26

2. Cardiac Arrest ──心停止 ········· 31

    Dialogue ········· 32

3. Respiratory Arrest ──呼吸停止 ········· 34

    Dialogue ········· 35

4. Hospital emergency procedures (anaphylaxisis) ········· 38
──病院救急医療（過敏症）

    Dialogue ········· 39

Relevant expressions and additional phrases ········· 43

   1) **Idiomatic expressions of negation**　否定を表す慣用表現

   2) **Idiomatic expressions of bare infinitive**
      原形不定詞の慣用表現

   3) **Link words (amplification)**　つなぎ言葉（増幅）

   4) **Compound medical words**　合成医学用語

   5) **Taking vital signs**　バイタルサインを調べる

Chapter III.　Prevention of lifestyle disease ········· 47
　　　　　　　生活習慣病の予防

1.　Definition of lifestyle disease ──生活習慣病の定義 ········· 47

Dialogue ········· 47

Relevant expressions and additional phrases ········· 50

   1) **Qualifier**　修飾（話しにあやをつける）

   2) **Time order**　時間的順序

2.　Dietary habits ──食習慣 ········· 51

Dialogue ········· 52

Relevant expressions and additional phrases ········· 62

   1) **Idiomatic parenthesis**　慣用的挿入句

   2) **Hyphenated words**　ハイフン連結用語

   3) **Infinitive and root verbs**　不定詞と原形動詞

3.　Smoking ──喫煙 ········· 63

Dialogue ········· 63

Relevant expressions and additional phrases ········· 67

   1) **Synergism and antagonism**　相乗効果・拮抗作用

   2) **Degree of morbidity**　罹患の程度

   3) **How to turn down softly**　丁寧な断り方

   4) **Periphrastic expressions**　婉曲表現

4.　Stress and Depression ──ストレスとうつ病 ········· 69

Dialogue ········· 70

Relevant expressions and additional phrases ·················· 73
- 1) Calendar　暦
- 2) Phrasal verbs　動詞句
- 3) Expression of feelings　感情表現
- 4) Faultfinding　揚げ足をとる

Chapter IV.　Suggestions based on laboratorytest results ·················· 77
検査値に基づくアドバイス

1. Hyperlipidemia due to obesity ──肥満による高脂血症 ·················· 77
Dialogue ·················· 78
Relevant expressions and additional phrases ·················· 85
- 1) Expression of numerical formula　数式の表現
- 2) Eating habits　食習慣

2. Type II diabetes due to lack of exercise ·················· 87
──運動不足によるII型糖尿病
Dialogue ·················· 88
Relevant expressions and additional phrases ·················· 93
- 1) Huge numbers　大きな数字
- 2) Function of organs　臓器の機能

3. Hyperuricemia due to excessive drinking ·················· 95
──過度の飲酒による高尿酸血症
Dialogue ·················· 96
Relevant expressions and additional phrases ·················· 105
- 1) Absence　休暇
- 2) Limit of patience　我慢の限界
- 3) Resignation　諦め
- 4) Know-how　コツ（秘策）
- 5) Common expressions of excretion　排泄の一般表現
- 6) Proverbs / sayings　諺・格言

Chapter V. Musculoskeletal Injuries ⋯⋯⋯⋯⋯⋯⋯⋯⋯⋯ 109
　　　　　　筋骨格損傷

1. Shoulder girdle injuries ──肩帯損傷 ⋯⋯⋯⋯⋯⋯⋯⋯⋯ 111

A. Dislocation and subluxation of the shoulder joint ⋯⋯⋯⋯⋯ 111
　　──肩関節の脱臼と亜脱臼

B. Dislocation of the acromiocravicular joint ⋯⋯⋯⋯⋯⋯⋯ 113
　　──肩鎖関節脱臼病

　1) Patient's complaints　患者の愁訴

　2) Radiographic examinations　X線検査

　3) Rehabilitation　リハビリテーション

C. Subluxation associated with glenoid labrum tear ⋯⋯⋯⋯⋯ 116
　　──関節唇の剥離に伴う亜脱臼

　1) Radiographic examinations

　2) Rehabilitation

2. Elbow injuries ──肘の損傷 ⋯⋯⋯⋯⋯⋯⋯⋯⋯⋯⋯⋯ 119

A. Tennis elbow (lateral epicondylitis) ⋯⋯⋯⋯⋯⋯⋯⋯⋯ 120
　　and Thrower's elbow (medial epicondylitis)
　　──テニス肘（外側上顆炎）と投球肘（内側上顆炎）

B. Loose bodies in the elbow joint (osteochondritis dissecans) ⋯⋯⋯ 121
　　──肘関節の遊離体（離断性骨軟骨炎）

　1) Patient's complaints

　2) Radiographic examinations

　3) Rehabilitation

3. Lumbar spine injuries ──腰痛 ⋯⋯⋯⋯⋯⋯⋯⋯⋯⋯⋯ 125

　1) Patient's complaints

　2) Radiographic examinations

　3) Radiographic findings

　4) Rehabilitation

4. Knee injuries ──膝関節部の損傷 ⋯⋯⋯⋯⋯⋯⋯⋯⋯⋯ 132

A. Knee joint ──膝関節 ⋯⋯⋯⋯⋯⋯⋯⋯⋯⋯⋯⋯⋯⋯ 134

　1) Radiographic examination

2）Rehabilitation
　B. Patella and patellofemoral joint ──膝蓋骨と膝蓋大腿関節 ············ 137
　　1）Patient's complaints
　　2）Radiographic examination
　　3）Rehabilitation
　Relevant expressions and additional phrases ······················ 140
　　1）Expressions of definitions　定義の表現
　　2）Geometric expressions　幾何学的表現

Chapter VI.　Debate and discussion ···················· 145
　　　　　　　ディベートと会議

1.　Debate ──ディベート ·· 145

Proposition 1: Medical stuff (MS) should have a fixed assignment position ··· 145
論題1：医療スタッフの職場は固定されるべきである

　　Constructive speech of the affirmative side　肯定側の基調演説
　　Cross-examination by the opposing side　反対側の反対尋問
　　Constructive speech of the opposing side　反対側の基調演説
　　Cross-examination by affirmative side　肯定側の反対尋問
　　Rebuttal speech of affirmative side　肯定側の反駁
　　Rebuttal speech of the opposing side　反対側の反駁

Proposition 2: Competitive market system should be introduced to hospital administration. ····································· 152
論題2．病院管理に競争原理を導入すべきである

　　Constructive speech of the affirmative side　肯定側の基調演説
　　Cross-examination by the opposing side　反対側の反対尋問
　　Constructive speech of the opposing side　反対側の基調演説
　　Cross-examination by the affirmative side　肯定側の反対尋問

Reference　参考

Debate terminology　ディベート用語

2. Brainstorming ──ブレーンストーミング ································ 158

    The issue : How to avoid careless errors
    議題：いかにして人的エラーを減らすか

    Relevant expressions and additional phrases ···················· 161

      1) Idiomatic phrases of debate　ディベートの慣用表現

      2) Idiomatic expressions of discussion　会議の慣用表現

      3) Idiomatic expressions for general assembly　総会の慣用表現

Chapter VII. International conference　国際会議 ············ 167

1. General session ──一般演題 ·· 167

    Title: Smoking among Health Science University students
        in Japan
    演題：日本の医療技術大学生の喫煙について

2. Special lecture ──特別公演 ··· 170

    Title: Computer-Based Patient Records in Digital Hospitals
    演題：デジタル病院における電子カルテ

    Relevant expressions and additional phrases ···················· 174

      1) Tips for an effective power point presentation
        パワーポイント発表

      2) key expressions for powerpoint slide projection and room lighting
        パワーポイントスライド発表と室内灯に関する重要表現

3. Key expressions for the chairperson ······························· 176
   ──司会者のための重要表現

      1) When time is running short　時間が足りなくなってきたとき

      2) Idiomatic expressions in a pressing situation
        とっさのときの慣用表現

      3) When no one asks Mr. M a question

4. At a special speech ──特別公演で ································· 177

      1) Introduction　紹介

      2) Ending remarks　終わりに

3) Presentation of certificate along with a gift
   贈呈品と認証の授与

5. Key expressions for discussion periods ·········· 178
——質疑応答のための重要表現

1) Asking for questions from the floor　会場からの質問を求める
2) Asking for partial clarification　ある部分の詳述を求める
3) Making a comment rather than raising a question
   質問というよりコメントを述べる
4) Asking about a comparison　比較を尋ねる
5) Directing the question to another speaker
   他の演者に質問を向ける
6) Asking for an answer with an example　具体例で答えてもらう
7) When you couldn't follow the question asked in English
   質問を理解でないとき

6. key expressions for speeches at a party or dinner ·········· 180
——歓迎パーティ用のスピーチの重要表現

1) A conference officer gives a welcoming address
   学会関係者による歓迎スピーチ
2) A participant gives an address in thanks　参加者の謝辞
3) Acting as a toastmaster (toastmistress)
   乾杯の音頭をあずかって

References 参照文献 ·········· 185

Example answer ·········· 188

Appendix ·········· 195

1 ANATOMICAL TERMS　解剖用語 ·········· 195
2 ANATOMICAL AND COMMON NAMES FOR PARTS OF THE BODY ·········· 198
   人体各部の解剖学的名称と一般名

3 KEY EXPRESSIONS ON THE SPOT ········· 202
その場での重要表現

    1. At the registration counter　受付で

    2. Directions to patients　患者さんへの指示

    3. Expressions of breathing　呼吸

    4. Preparation for dressing or undressing　更衣の準備

    5. Before and after an examination　検査の前後

    6. Nursing care　看護処置

    7. Cold and pollen allergy　風邪と花粉症

    8. Trauma and generative symptoms　外傷と退行性の症状

    9. Patient's complaints and symptoms　患者の症状と愁訴

   10. Expressions of pain　痛みの表現

4 THE CONSTRUCTION OF ENGLISH ········· 209
構文別英会話集

    1. Causative verbs　使役動詞

    2. Subjunctive mood　仮定法

    3. Inanimate subject　物主構文

    4. Comparison　比較

    5. Insertion and ellipsis　挿入と省略

    6. Adverbial phrases　副詞句

    7. Inversions　倒置構文

5 100 SELECTED IDIOMATIC EXPRESSIONS ········· 213
慣用表現100選

6 COFFEE BREAK VOCABULARY　歓談用語句集 ········· 220

著者略歴

Chapter I.

Interaction with patients
患者接遇法

1. Building mutual reliance —— 信頼関係の構築

Dealing effectively with clinical situations involves several skills and a professional attitude. One of these skills is the ability to show empathy, being sensitive to the needs of others that allows you to meet their needs constructively, rather than merely sympathizing, or reacting to their distress. Understanding and compassion are accompanied by an **objective detachment**[*1] that enables you to provide an appropriate response. It is also very useful for cultivating the skill to **be assertive**[*2]. Expressions of aggression involve anger or hostility, whereas assertion is a calm, firm expression of feelings or opinions. In dealing with patients who are reluctant to cooperate, **pleasant assertiveness**[*3] is the attitude that is most productive in **obtaining compliance**[*4]. Such patients will **place** their **confidence in**[*5] medical personnel only if their expectations of a professional person are being met. With this in mind, you can be less **judgmental**[*6] about specific behaviors and face the patient directly. Assertiveness does not mean arrogance. **Looking down on**[*7] adults or treating them **impersonally**[*8] diminishes their **self-esteem**[*9] and raises feelings of resentment. Such feelings diminish a patient's ability to understand and follow directions, prevent retention of information, and may hinder recovery. Everyone we meet receives some impression of who we are. Outward appearance is also as important as behavioral appearance. Medical personnel should wear uniforms that present a neat appearance. The appearance of the examination room is equally important. An untidy, cluttered room does not reflect respect for patients.

Notes: *1 客観的で公平な態度, *2 きっぱりと指示をする, *3 小気味よい命令, *4 応諾を得る, *5 ～に信頼を置く, *6 主観的に, *7 見下した態度で物を言う, *8 物のように, *9 自尊心

Dialogue

Situation: A nursing unit is having a Team Care meeting on the subject of how medical staff should interact with patients by asking opinions from patient's families.　看護グループが"チーム医療会議"を開き，患者の家族を招待して意見交換を行っている

Leader: A good way to understand **what** patient care is **all about** is to ask oneself, "How would I want to be treated if I were the patient?" However, it's not as easy as you would think to always **put** yourself **in the** patient's **shoes**.　ペイシェント・ケアとは**一体何であるのか**／立場に身を置く

So, today, we invited patient's families, instead of patients themselves because they would hesitate to express themselves frankly, to give us some opinions as to what family members usually ask healthcare providers.

Family A: Please, let us hear your ideas. Try to think back to a time when you were a patient walking into a medical facility for the first time. What did you want or expect from medical personnel?

Nurse A: If I stand back and look at this question **from** a patient's **perspective**, I might **come up with** the expectation of being treated with **compassion** and **empathy**.　立場になってみる／思いつく／深い同情と共感をもって

Nurse B: I would like to **be listened to carefully**, and receive undivided **immediate** attention.　傾聴してもらう／隔てのない**即座**な対応を受ける

Nurse C: I would want to be provided with efficient and effective care.

Leader: These **sound like** simple and logical expectations. Maybe they are, but to accomplish them takes a lot of knowledge and practice. As you enter a department as a patient, you'll **appreciate** the extra effort it takes to provide the best patient care in the department.　一見容易に思える／特別な計らいに**感謝する**

Nurse D: Patient care includes **all the comments** we just heard. One must take care to observe, evaluate and assess changes in patient conditions, since such conditions might be the **deciding factor** in avoiding a **life-threatening emergency**.　ペイシェント・ケアは，私たちがいま聞いた**すべての意見**を含む／**緊急状態**にならないようにする**重要な指標**となる

Nurse E: Patient care starts with knowing about a patient's history, which allows med-

	ical staff to give the patient individual and thoughtful attention. All of these skills **aid in the assistance of** patients and their personal needs.　患者さんたち，さらに個々の要望に応えることに役立つ
Leader:	The first contact with a patient generally starts with a self-introduction. What else do you do when you address a patient?
Nurse A:	It reminds me of an early stage of my studies at school. We students recited phrases **in unison**, saying "**Break the ice**," "Introduce yourself to the patient," "**Make eye contact**," "Smile," and "**Use their first and last name**."　学生のころ，「口火を切ること（何かひとこと言って相手の凍りついた心を和らげる）」，「目を合わせること」，「同時に氏名を呼ぶこと」と斉唱した
Nurse B:	I think it is good manner to maintain eye contact with a patient, but we should not forget to smile while speaking. This is important **nonverbal communication** to help **alleviate** a patient's fear.　言語によらないコミュニケーション／和らげる
Nurse B:	I noticed that small talk with a patient after the greeting certainly can **break the ice**. I always try to avoid **heavy subjects** such as religion and private affairs; **but** am often **at a loss** to select a suitable subject when it's a rainy day. I can't use the stereotyped expression, "It's fine today, isn't it?" Is there any appropriate expression?　気楽にさせる／差障りのある言葉を避ける（i.e. taboo phrases：禁句）／戸惑う
Leader:	Our staff usually **share** what they are doing when they meet patients. Do you think what the staff are doing is always **an agreeable topic to bring up?**　同じようなことを言う／常に言行が一致していますか
Family A:	I appreciate staff members kindness. If I dared to add a suggestion, I would ask that you always call a patient by his/her full name, **not doing away** with the first name. The other day, the **wrong** patient went into a room instead of my mother because his last name **happened to be the same** as my mother's.　名前を省かないで／間違った患者さん／偶然一致した
Family B:	Most patients must have come to the hospital with some health problem. Moreover, they are scared of staff walking around in white coats and of the **stark** hospital **environment**. Would you mind giving them a word of encouragement when you pass them in the hall even though I know you are always busy?　病院独特の息苦しい雰囲気
Leader:	Thank you for your frank opinions and suggestions. I understand we should

try to read a patient's mind more carefully. The last topic is how we can **live up to the confidence** a patient places in us. Any other comments?
〜に与えられた期待に応える

Family B: I am sorry to say that my father **would have been** more cooperative if someone **had told** him what was going to be done to him before his examination. （付録：仮定法過去参照）

Leader: I agree with you. **By doing so**, we could have helped relieve his anxieties. そうすることにより（つなぎ言葉参照）

Family C: I would like you to take a calm (**assertive**) attitude in **winning** a patient's **confidence**. If health providers **act timidly** in front of a patient, I think it reflects a lack of confidence in their skill; and the patient will doubt their capability. I don't think this kind of patient care will enable a patient to **recover** his/her health **earlier than when treated properly**.　　冷静（決断的）な態度／患者さんの信頼を得る／おどおどする／〜より効果が少ない（i.e. be less beneficial）

Family C: I know you are trying to interact with each patient on **an equal footing**. However, I occasionally see someone who speaks politely, but is actually impolite under the cover of politeness. My grandpa was treated as if he was a child, which **hurt** his **feelings**.　　同じ目線で（目線を合わせる参照）／慇懃無礼な言葉で／感情を害した

Family D: My father was treated as if he was a sack of potatoes after he was transported to the emergency area. It's **too much** to call him "a whale" by name **simply because** he is stout. He was **sober enough** to understand how he was treated. I hope all medical staff **behave themselves** when conversing among colleagues.　　身体が大きいからと言って，名前の代わりに鯨と呼ぶのはあんまりだ／どのように取り扱われているかを充分に判断ができた／正しくふるまう

Family E: It's not a direct request to you, but when you providers ask us for **informed consent**, please explain the possible hazards in an **easy-to-understand way**, not using too much medical **jargon**.　　納得診療（あるいは"十分な説明に基づく同意"と訳される）／わかりやすい方法で／医学専門用語を使わずに

Leader: We understand how improper speech and behavior can causes a negative reaction from patients. We must take considerate care toward each patient's earliest recovery showing a positive attitude, because **"the mind rules the body"** as they say. I'll bring up the issues discussed here at the coming hospital meeting. Thank you so much for your frank opinions. We **have learned** a lot, today.　　"病は気から" と言われるように／大変参考になりました

Quiz

- **A.** What kinds of skills are necessary for dealing effectively with clinical situations?
- **B.** Describe "pleasant assertiveness."
- **C.** What problems can an attitude of arrogance cause?
- **D.** What role do outward appearances play in communication?
- **E.** What expectations do patients and their families generally have of healthcare providers?
- **F.** How should you "break the ice" with patients?

Answers

- **A.** One necessary skill is the ability to show empathy, being sensitive to the needs of others. Also the skills of understanding and compassion, accompanied by an objective detachment enables one to provide appropriate responses. It is also very useful to cultivate the skill to be pleasantly assertive.
- **B.** It is the calm, firm expression of feelings or opinions in a pleasant manner. In dealing with patients who are reluctant to cooperate, pleasant assertiveness is the attitude that is most productive in obtaining compliance.
- **C.** Arrogance, or looking down on patients and treating them impersonally, diminishes their self-esteem and raises feelings of resentment. Such feelings diminish a patient's ability to understand and follow directions, prevent retention of information, and may hinder recovery.
- **D.** Everyone we meet receives some impression of who we are by our outward appearance. Medical personnel should wear uniforms that present a neat appearance to reflect professionalism. The appearance of the examination room is equally important. An untidy, cluttered room does not reflect respect for patients.
- **E.** They expect to be treated with compassion and empathy, listened to carefully, and provided with efficient and effective care.
- **F.** Introduce yourself to the patient, make eye contact, smile, and use their first and last names.

Relevant expressions and additional phrases

1) Subjunctive Mood　　仮定法

Consider how you **would be** treated if you **were** a patient.　　もしあなたが患者だったら

He **would have been** more cooperative if you **had told** him what was going to be done to him.

Treat patients with the same concern that you **would** appreciate if you **were** ill.
あなたが病気だったとき，ありがたいと思う気配り

2) Causative Verbs　　使役動詞

・The patient will feel at ease if you relieve him of his anxiety.　　安心する
　We **made** him **feel** at ease.　　安心させた
・Breaking the ice using small talk will melt a patient's heart.
　We **had** him **relax**.　　リラックスさせた（人＋原形）
・The patient felt relieved because you set him at ease.
　Your considerate attitude **had** his mind **relieved**.　　ほっとさせた（物＋過去分詞）　＠通常会話では〜relieved him.
・Most patients are scared of unfamiliar surroundings in a hospital.
　Ambulances going in and out **caused** them to **feel** uneasy.　　不安にさせた

3) Collective Nouns　　集合名詞

・staff / personnel（uncountable：不可算）・medical professionals（countable：可算）

The team consists of 5 staff members.

The team consists of 3 different health staff (different staff members, such as an RN, RT, OT, etc.)

The medical staff make a great effort when working in team medicine.

Half of the hospital personnel are women.　cf. He is hospital personnel.

Professionals are personnel who are not easily substituted by another person.

＠ I hope this letter finds you and your family in good health.　　手紙の結語（あなたとご家族の皆様のご多幸を）

4) Expressions for mutual reliance　　信頼関係に関する表現

- 信頼する　　put（place）confidence in（a person）
- 信頼に応える　　live up to the patient's expectations

  e.g. come up to ~ , comply with ~ , meet ~ , answer ~ , satisfy ~
- 信頼を裏切る　　betray a patient's trust

  e.g. fall short of ~ , run counter to ~ , fail to meet ~ , let down ~
- 信頼関係を結ぶ　　build rapport with（a person）

It is important for us to **gain** the patient's confidence and **relieve** his anxiety.　信頼を得る／心配を和らげる

We need to **live up to** the confidence a patient **places**（puts）in us.　　患者さんの**期待に応える**

Rapport is a relationship based on trust and empathy.　　ラポルトとは信頼と感情移入に基づいた対人間関係である。

Empathy is referred to as a mental entering into the feeling of a person. For example, a reader is so deeply immersed in the story that he / she unconsciously plays a part of the hero or heroine in mind. It differs from actions following compassion or sympathy **in that** empathetic actions rise above one's reason.　　感情移入とは，相手と立場を共有することを指す。読者が小説に読みふけると，主人公の立場になりきるのがその例である。この感情が理性を超えたものである**という点で**同情と異なる。

5) Expressions for a cautious attitude　　慎重な態度に関する表現

Prior to the examination, give a patient a clear explanation of the procedure to **ensure** his / her cooperation.　　患者さんの協力を**確証する**

Call him by his **last**（**surname** or **family**）**name** and **first name**（**given name**）as well.　　**苗字**だけでなく**名前**も呼ぶ

You should always call a patient by his / her full name, **not doing away with** the first name.　　省略しないで

Be sure not to call in a **wrong** patient **by accident** by neglecting his / her first name.　間違って別の患者さんを呼ぶ

　　e.g. I'm very sorry. I called the **wrong number**.　　間違い電話でした

6) Taking accountability　　説明責任を果たす（Give と Take の混同を避ける）

Be sure the patient **has given** informed consent before the medical treatment.

患者さんの同意を**得ている**か

We must take every precaution in **getting** consent from a patient when the treatment involves a risk.   同意を**得る**とき

We should **take accountability** for the treatment **by giving** them a clear explanation of the fact that the benefits **outweigh possible risks by a reasonable margin**.

説明責任を負う／詳しく説明して／予期される危険をある程度のゆとりをもって上回る

2. Interacting with children and elderly patients
——子供と老齢患者への対応

Children are more likely than adults to respond negatively to the strange surroundings and machines of the hospital environment. A professional approach, **coupled with***1 warm reassurance, promotes a more positive attitude in both children and **adolescents***2. A child's first impression of you will decide what his / her attitude will be for the following examination. Children usually judge whether or not you are a person who they can trust and will **protect them***3 when they see you enter the waiting room. When **venipuncture***4 is necessary, never **trick** the child **into***5 having it by saying, "It won't hurt you at all." If you do this, he will become very unwilling to allow **anything similar to happen***6 again. On the other hand, you need not unnecessarily tell him the whole truth beforehand. Just encourage him to say "Would you be a good boy and have this shot?" Many poor attitudes toward health care shown by adults may be **traced back to***7 a lack of sensitive care by health professionals in the adult's early years. Many adults show **higher blood pressure***8 than usual when sitting in front of a staff member who wears **a white coat**.

Elderly patients also require special attention because of the physical problems that often **accompany aging***9. A typical attitude of aging is a tendency to **proceed at one's own pace***10, both mentally and physically. Most elderly patients do not respond well to feeling pushed or hurried. They are **reluctant to surrender their independence***11. Never treat them **in too condescending a fashion***12, and always allow them to do what they can for themselves. It's true that this will **require more patience***13 than doing everything for the patient.

Notes: *1 暖かい勇気付けと**相俟**って（cf. couple statement with action）言行を一致さ

せる，＊2 青春期（成人前の）患者，＊3 **味方か否かを判断する**，＊4 静脈（穿刺）注射（shot），＊5 だまして〜させる，＊6 同じような検査で，＊7 子どものころに受けた医療従事者の配慮のなさによる，＊8 白衣高血圧，＊9 加齢に伴う（cf. aging process）老化現象，＊10 マイペースで行動する，＊11 自律性を失うことを嫌がる，＊12 恩着せがましい態度，＊13 〜より我慢がいる

Dialogue

Situation: A Junior staff member (J. staff) is asking a senior staff member (S. staff) how to interact with aged and pediatric patients.
新入スタッフ（J. staff）が先輩（S. staff）に，高齢者と子どもの患者さんに対する接し方を教わっている。

Case 1

J. staff: I had to do another exam on him because he responded to my call for another patient with the same name.

S. staff: Haven't I told you that you should always call a patient by their full name?

J. staff: That's what I did.

S. staff: Okay, now listen. An elderly person may not hear you correctly. If you merely call Mr. So-and-so, some patient who has been waiting for a long time may reply. Such a long wait under strain often tends to put the patient in a sort of **mentally incapacitated state**.
長い間緊張して待っていると，老齢患者さんは往々にして**極度ののぼせ状態**になる。
Be careful about the elderly who come here alone. They may have some degree of **senile dementia**. Anyway, you mustn't only rely on the patient to tell you his name, but rather check with the **chart** to confirm his identity before beginning a procedure.
ある程度の**老人性痴呆症**／患者さんの応答だけに頼らず**カルテ**で氏名を確認する

J. staff: Even when we're in a hurry or maybe preoccupied?

S. staff: Yes. And, never forget to the term, "Break the ice" which you learned at school. When you deal with a patient who appears confused, ask him where he was born and how many grandchildren he has. **Long-term memory is frequently still clear** when the patient can no longer recall what was served for breakfast. While conversing with him and **asking questions about his**

past, you'll find he will cooperate much better in following your directions. 今朝の朝食が何であったかを思い出せなくても，**遠い過去の記憶は確かなことが多い**／会話を交わすときに**時代を辿って質問を行う**と，患者さんがどれほど指示に従えるかがわかる

Case 2

S. staff: You shouldn't have **taken your** eyes **off** that child. At that age, a child tends to **run** desperately **after** his mother if she leaves him. In some cases, this has caused a child to fall off the table and fracture a bone. **It's consoling to think that** at least this child was not injured at all.
目を離す／必死に**後を追う**／怪我のなかったのが**不幸中の幸い**

J. staff: The child always cries when he sees me. I **can't manage** him alone. He is too **spoiled**.　手に負えない／とんでもない**甘えん坊**

S. staff: Listen to me. A sick child is likely to **be cross**, so you have to **see to it that** he doesn't have to wait a long time. You'd better call him in as quickly as possible, even if **it's out of turn**. The other patients usually won't mind if you tell them the reason.　むずかる／図ってあげる／順番どおりでない

J. staff: That's what I always do with him.

S. staff: You should have **made friends with** him before the exam. When you find a child that is **supposed to be** your patient, smile at him and say "hello" **at his eye level** whenever you see him. You will find that this is most effective when you've approached the child to make friends. During the exam use **his first name**. Try to find out what the child is called at home by asking him, "What does your mom call you at home?"　友達になる（必ず複数）／当然あなたの患者／（膝を折って）その子の**目の高さで**／**愛称で**

Moreover, the child's mother came and complained to me **furiously** about the treatment her son received when he had the contrast examination. You shouldn't have allowed him to leave the room with barium around his mouth and on his hands. You should always **return** the child to his mother **washed up** and **clean**. His mother will judge the **rest of our work by this single instance**, and form opinions about the quality of our department and hospital.　血相を変えて／（口を）拭いてきれいにして返す／**一事を万事として**

J. staff: He **broke free of** me. But I know now that I should have been his friend.
振りきって逃げた

S. staff: Okay. I'll go and apologize to his mother telling her what you said and that you've **learned** your **lesson**. あなたの言い分と戒めの気持ちを

Quiz
A. When giving a child a shot, what is the cardinal rule to remember?
B. Why do many adults have a poor attitude toward health care?
C. Why are many elderly patients hesitant to receive assistance?
D. What technique is useful for handling elderly patients who seem confused?
E. Why must medical staff be sure not to take their eyes off pediatric patients?
F. What is the secret to successfully dealing with pediatric patients?

Answers
A. Never trick the child into having it by saying, "It won't hurt you at all."
B. Such an attitude can often be traced back to a lack of sensitive care by health professionals in the adult's childhood.
C. They feel reluctant to surrender their independence. (Note: Never treat them in too condescending a fashion, and always allow them to do what they can for themselves. It's true that this will require more patience than doing everything for them.)
D. When you deal with a patient who appears confused, ask him where he was born and how many grandchildren he has. Long-term memory is frequently still clear when the patient can no longer recall what was served for breakfast. While conversing with him and asking questions about his past, you'll find he will cooperate much better in following your directions.
E. At certain ages, a child tends to run desperately after his mother if she leaves him. In some cases, this has caused an accident such as the child falling off the table and fracturing a bone.
F. Be friends with them as early on as possible. When you find a child that is supposed to be your patient, smile at him and say "hello" at his eye level whenever you see him. You will find that this is most effective when you've approached the child to make friends. During the exam use his first name.

Relevant expressions and additional phrases

1) Expressions of behavior   態度に関する表現
Never **look down on** him   見下す

We shouldn't talk to patients **with a superior tone of voice**.　　威張った口調で
Never treat an elderly patient **in a condescending fashion**.　　（優越感からわざと）
へりくだった態度で
　　i.e. in a ***politely insolent*** manner.　　慇懃無礼な態度で
Face the patient and **make direct eye contact** as he / she speaks and responds.
まっすぐ相手の目を見る（場合によっては脅迫的になる）
Try not to treat a patient like a sack of potatoes.　　物扱いする
a guinea pig.　　モルモットのように扱う
　@実験動物として使われるモルモット（marmot）はまったく別の動物である。
　e.g. For **clinical trials**, the doctor got extraordinary money from a pharmaceutical company, turning patients into **guinea pigs**. (Of Mice and Men：CBS)　　その医師は治験で，患者をモルモット代わりにして製薬会社から大金をもらった

2) Understanding patient's physical and mental conditions
患者の様態・気持ちを察する
Do you **need** help? You look **out of condition**.　　どうかしましたか／具合が悪そうですが
　cf. He may have something wrong **with** his stomach.
We should **take** his feelings **to heart**.　　気持ちを察する
　〈or〉We should **understand** how the patient is feeling.
　〈or〉We must **read** the patient's mind.
If we lack consideration for a patient, it will **hurt** his / her feelings　　患者の感情を害する

3) Psychological and physical aspects of eye level　　心理的な目線と物理的な目線
Speak to children **at their own eye level** by lowering yourself **to your knees** when children are short.　　小さな子どもの場合は膝をついて，同じ目の高さで話す
Talk to a patient **on an equal footing**.　　同じ目線で，患者さんと話す

4) Difference between Watch and See　　Watch と See の違い
　・Watch：look with attention　　気をつけて見る
　・See：perceive with the eyes　　目で見る
See if the patient can feel at home.　　患者さんがリラックスできるか確認する

See that we called in the **right patient**.　　本人を呼んだか確認する
We should always **watch** him.　　見守る
　　　　　　　　keep our eyes **on** him.
　　　　　　　　pay close **attention to** him.
　cf. Try not to **take** your eyes **off** him.　　目を離す

5) A state of mental incapacitation　　のぼせの状態
go to pieces　　自制心を失って心がばらばらになる
The pitcher **went to pieces** after filling the bases.　　満塁でピッチャーはあがってしまった。〈or〉With the bases loaded, the pitcher went to pieces.
　@ get nervous（のぼせとは異なり）神経質になる，緊張する
He got **nervous** before the examination.　　検査の前に**緊張した**

3. Dealing with a terminally ill patient
――末期患者への対応

　The terminally ill patient is usually in an emotional state of grieving. Dr. Elizabeth Kubler-Ross points out that grief is an emotional readjustment to a new way of experiencing life and cannot be accomplished all at once. She identifies five phases of the grieving process in turn: **Denial, Anger, Bargaining, Depression** and **Acceptance**[*1]. You need to know that the phases listed here are in general, and the time required to pass from one phase to the next varies with individuals. However, it will improve your ability to care for the terminally ill patient if you assess him prior to beginning care to determine which phase of the **grieving process**[*2] he may be going through.

　It is natural that family members accompany patients to their appointments and visit them during **hospital admission**[*3]. You will have to deal with family members who eagerly await the results of a diagnostic procedure. If the patient is **grief-stricken**[*4], you may need to provide instructions to a family member regarding **preparation or follow-up care**[*5]. Be sure you are speaking to the person who will **actually assist the patient**[*6], since important **information can be lost**[*7] when it is passed from person to person.

Notes: *1 否認, 怒り, 契約, 抑うつ, 受容の5段階, *2 悲しみの過程, *3 入院
　　　cf. hospital discharge：退院, *4 悲しみに打ち負ける, *5 検査前後の注意事項
　　　*6 信頼できる介添者か, *7 守秘義務が破られる

Dialogue

Situation: A Senior staff member (S. staff) is teaching a junior staff member (J. staff) about how her junior should have coped with each case.　先輩スタッフが後輩に，各々のケースについてどのような対応をとるべきだったか指導している

Case 1

S. staff: You shouldn't have talked so much with that patient about her individual case.

J. staff: What else could I do to cheer her up? She desperately wanted to **unburden herself**.　（気持ちの）**負担を軽くする**

S. staff: You have a point there. But **what if** she tells her **doctor in charge** what you've told her? If his remarks are inconsistent with yours, the patient will not know what to think and the doctor will **be at a loss** to explain the discrepancies. Moreover, she could have talked to other patients who may not have been told "You'll be alright." And the other patients may **take it for granted** that their illness must be malignant.　〜したらどうする／主治医，cf. referring doctor（a doctor who refers a patient or makes a referral: 紹介医）／困ってしまう／（間違って）思い込む

J. staff: Do you mean we should just close the door on conversation and reassuring the patient?

S. staff: No, that's not what I mean. I mean it's a matter of method. It's always best to speak in general. For example, "There aren't as many malignant cases as you think." You have to be especially careful not to be trapped when a person asks a **leading question**. She may say something like "I've got to take it easy **now that** my doctor has told me frankly that my case is malignant." If you hear this, never say "Don't worry, I hear that yours is in an early stage." The patient will then know what it is for sure.　誘導質問に引っかからないように注意する／お医者さんが正直に癌だと言ってくださったので

J. staff: How should I respond to then?

S. staff: Just listen or say something **non-committal** like "We always try our best, whatever the patient's illness may be." An **expression of concern** can show empathy.　差し障りのないこと／関心を示せば共感が伝わる

J. staff:	I first told her to refer her inquiry directly to the doctor. But I thought it would hurt her feelings if I **turned down** any inquiries **flatly**. 　どんな質問にも素っ気なく断る
S. staff:	First of all, you should have clarified yourself before you **went too far** to turn back. Tell the patient that you are not allowed to say anything about the results. **The thing is** how we can **maintain confidentiality of individual information** before the doctor has really disclosed the truth. 深入りしすぎて後戻りできない／問題は〜／個人情報の守秘義務を守る

Case 2

J. staff:	I really **got mad** at the patient. He was upset and **took it out** on me. 本当に頭にくる／逆上して八つ当たりする
S. staff:	Come now, calm down. You know what they say "**Sound mind, sound body.**" **The flip side of this is also true**. That patient is also mentally upset. 健全な身体に健全な精神が宿るというが逆もまた真なり
J. staff:	Don't you think it's **wrong for him** to shout at someone just because he is in a bad mood?　誰彼となく怒鳴るのは**あんまりだ**
S. staff:	**There's more to it than that**. I think he has fallen into the stage that we would call "anger."　そんな単純なものではない
J. staff:	What would that be?
S. staff:	It is one of the stages, well, of dying. Remember when he first came here? He wouldn't accept his illness. He was always saying that the test results must be wrong or he was sent here by mistake. That was the first stage, which we call "denial." Once he knows he can not deny the truth any longer, **he blows his top** shouting "Why does this have to happen to me and not someone else?" This anger will be directed at anybody **irrespective of who it** is. It is said to be caused by complex feelings mingled with envy and jealousy. 「どうして自分だけがこんな目に」と**感情を爆発させる**／この怒りは**誰彼構わずに向けられる**
J. staff:	You mean this is the stage he is at now?
S. staff:	Yes. **As time goes by**, he will shift to the third stage, called "bargaining." He will plead for his life saying, "I will do anything I can if you save my life." At this stage, even an atheist will try to bargain with God, **grasping at straws**, and with anyone that's treating him in the hope that he might be treated in a special way with a secret technique or medicine if he is cooperative.

そのうちに（長期的）"契約"と呼ばれる段階に入る／無神論者であっても，藁をもつかむ気持ちで神に誓う

J. staff: Can you believe that his rage will calm down **in time**? 　怒りは**まもなく**おさまる

S. staff: There are always exceptions, of course; but **by and large** patients follow these stages. I think it is better than treating a patient in depression. After the anger stage comes "depression." This stage comes after the patient has given up all hope of escape. 　例外はあるが，**大体は**この過程を辿る

J. staff: What can we do for such a patient?

S. staff: Nothing, but just show him you care and are doing your best in treating him. You're asking how we can cheer him up with words; but, in reality, we can't. Any attempt **would only be in vain**. 　（言葉で）元気づけてもむなしくなるだけ

Don't talk like the patient is going to be fine. Such responses tend to block communication and may **be insulting** to a patient who has long since passed the stage of denial. 　そのような応答では会話が途絶え，否認の過程をとっくに過ぎた患者さんを**侮辱**することになる

J. staff: Then no verbal communication at all?

S. staff: Remember that the patient is **not necessarily seeking a direct verbal response**. What is needed is a friendly, **supportive listener**. It will encourage the patient to keep talking so that he starts feeling better automatically. 患者さんは**必ずしも直接的な返答を求めているのではない**／求めているのは好意的で，**精神的に支援してくれる聞き役**である

J. staff: How can I be a supportive listener?

S. staff: **Just rephrase the patient's remarks by saying**, for example, "Oh, you are feeling tired of living" or " You're feeling better today." Don't be afraid to get **involved or show that you care**. 　ただ患者さんの言葉を反復しなさい。たとえば，「そうですか，生きるのに疲れたのですか」とか「今日は気分がよいのですか」とか。**関わる**ことや，真正面から対応することにおじけてはいけない

J. staff: That's just the opposite of how I've responded so far. I am at a loss.

S. staff: But this stage is not the end. Most patients will **get over** the despair and calmly prepare for death with dignity. 　絶望を**乗り越えて**，威厳をもって静かに死を覚悟する

There will be no anger and no depression anymore. This is the final stage which is called "acceptance." If you closely watch for these stages, you will be enabled to **interact with the patient more objectively and less emotionally**.　感情的でなく客観的に患者さんと接触できる

It will help to keep all of this advice **in mind**. If you don't, you may **find it too sad to work with** terminally ill patients.　このことを覚えておくと役に立つ／さもないと末期患者と接触するのが辛すぎて勤まらなくなる

Quiz

A. What is Dr. Elizabeth Kubler-Ross's definition of grief?
B. What are the five phases of the grieving process?
C. When providing instructions to a patient's family member, what must you be sure to do?
D. Why should medical staff be careful about speaking too much about a particular patient's condition with the patient?
E. What kind of reaction might a patient have in the "denial" phase?
F. What happens in the "bargaining" phase?

Answers

A. It is an emotional readjustment to a new way of experiencing life and cannot be accomplished all at once.
B. Denial, Anger, Bargaining, Depression and Acceptance
C. You must be sure to speak directly to the person who will actually assist the patient, since important information can be lost when it is passed from person to person.
D. Such comments may conflict with what the doctor in charge or other medical staff have told the patient causing confusion or lack of trust.
E. Such a patient won't accept his illness making comments like, "The test results must be wrong" or "I was sent here by mistake."
F. The patient usually pleads for his life saying something like, "I will do anything I can if you save my life." At this stage, even an atheist will try to bargain with God, grasping at straws, and with anyone that's treating him in the hope that he might be treated in a special way with a secret technique or medicine if he is cooperative.

Relevant expressions and additional phrases

1) Expressions of anger　　怒りの表現
He **got angry at** me.　　怒った
He was **upset at** me.　or, He got **mad at** me.　　私に対して逆上した
He **took the anger out on** me.　　私に八つ当たりした
He **blew his top**.　　切れた

2) Psychological leading　　心理的誘導
She may **trick** you into **telling** the truth.　　かまをかける
The truth is, she hadn't heard it from the doctor.　　本当は医者に知らされていなかった（注：Be 動詞の後のコンマはなくてもよい）
Never **trick** the child into your **giving** him / her a shot by saying that it won't hurt at all.　　だまして〜する　or, **fool** one into 〜ing,
Try to talk him into your giving a shot by saying "Be a good boy."　　説得して〜させる　or, **coax** one into 〜ing　　なだめて〜させる

3) Flat and involved attitudes　　素っ気ない態度と深入りし過ぎた態度
He **refused it flatly**　　露骨に拒絶する
＠ I left the cap off the bottle and it **went flat**.　　瓶のふたを空けっぱなしにしていたら（炭酸飲料の）気が抜けた（素っ気ない味）
There's nothing more to say. That's **all there is to it**.　　もうなにも言うことはありません。ただそれだけのことです
You've gone too far past the **point of no return**.　　深入りしてもう戻れない
＠ The airplane has reached the point of no return on the runway.　　飛行機はその点まで滑走したら離陸以外に道はない
You may **get caught up in the emotion** of the situation and **find it very difficult to see him**.　　感情に流されて，見るに忍びない

4) Passing time　　時間的経過
As time goes by, he will change his mind.　　時が経てば
＠ "時の流れるまま" 映画カサブランカの主題歌
We can see his behavior **changes over time**.　　経過観察をしましょう
Leave him alone **for the time being**.　　しばらくはそのままにしてあげなさい

He will settle down **in time**.　　そのうちに落ち着く

4. Stress management
　　　　　　　　　　　　　　　　　　　　　──ストレス管理

　Any situation that disturbs everyday activities imposes stress. Most health care involves some stress, and the hospital environment often proves stressful to both patients and medical staff. This is especially true in crisis situations when speed is a factor or when disagreement exists about what should be done in team medicine. Stress is usually higher than ever when working in an emergency room. Sometimes dealing with families can be especially difficult in an emotionally charged situation. They experience fear and anxiety, and these feelings may be displaced to the closest professional person. Fear frequently **engenders anger**[*1]. If you can understand aggressive demands for service and attention **as being an expression of fear**[*2], you can concentrate on **reassuring** rather than responding with anger **yourself**[*3].

　Students majoring in allied health sciences in the USA discuss the matter before they go out for clinical practice. They are asked how to cope with each case after watching a TV program that includes trouble cases they may encounter in a hospital. We must learn how to calm a patient and their family down even under crucial stressful conditions. A popular method for self-control or anger control is Rational Emotive Behavior Therapy (**REBT**) [*4] initiated by Dr. Albert Ellis.

　Dr Ellis, a pioneer in the field of psychotherapy, states that REBT has three main constructive philosophies. The first is **USA**[*5] (Unconditional Self Acceptance) where you accept yourself as you are. The second is **UOA**[*6] (Unconditional Other Acceptance) where you never damn other people. You may damn what they do; but you never tell someone they are totally no good, they deserve to die, etc. And, the third is **ULA**[*7] (Unconditional Life Acceptance) where you don't damn the world. You accept the fact that things are often very bad, deplorable, sad, but it's not the end of the world. Life goes on.

　REBT teaches that one can, and should, take responsibility for one's own emotions. That is, one can **select** one's own **emotion**[*8] or reaction before acting it out (rage or calmness) even when the other person, for example a patient, makes unreasonable complaints. Thus, a situation never brings about an action directly. There are two steps between a **situation** and **reaction**[*9]. Therefore you need to take responsibility for your emotions.

Notes: ＊1 怒りを誘発する， ＊2 恐怖の表れとして， ＊3 怒りでなく**自信をもって対応**

する，＊4 認知行動療法，＊5 無条件の自己受容，＊6 無条件の他者受容，＊7 無条件の状況受容，＊8（行動する前に，激怒するか鎮まるかの）感情を選択できる，＊9 **状況と反応**（の間に2段階がある）

Dialogue

Case 1

Situation: A staff member who received the same kind of complaint in two different cases offended the first patient's attendant, but took a positive attitude towards the second one.　2人の患者さんから同様な苦情を受けたスタッフが，最初は患者介添者の怒りを買ったが，2度目には前向きな態度を示す

Bad example: **Yielding to patient's provocation**　患者さんの挑発に乗ってしまう

Attendant: How long will you make my father wait! We've been here for thirty minutes. **On top of that**, a person who came after my father was called in before him.　おまけに，後からの人が先に呼ばれるなんて

Staff: Sorry. His **number** will be called soon. Anyway, the order is **subject to** patient condition.　すぐに**順番**がくる／**順番**は患者さんの状態により**変更になる**

Attendant: You shouldn't make him wait without any explanation.

Staff: We **have been tied up** with our immediate work. And an **in-patient** was sent here when her condition **took a sudden** turn for the worse.　急用で**手が空かなかった**／あの**入院患者**さんの様態が**急変したので**

Attendant: How long does it take for you to tell us of a schedule change beforehand? Anybody would have understood if they had been given an explanation earlier.

Staff: You don't realize that we have too many emergency cases for such a small work force.

Attendant: That's no excuse for a lack of courtesy!

Good example

　Selecting positive behavior based on the following five steps of REBT　REBT（認知行動療法）の5段階のステップに基づき前向きな行動をとる

　1 **Identify negative thinking**　マイナス思考を認識する

　I'm **becoming** emotional.　自分も感情的に**なりかけている**

　Emotionally-charged behavior always **gives rise to** an escalation of the tension level.　緊張度を増すことになる

2. **Deny negative thinking**　　マイナス思考を否定する
   Let me **try** to see the matter from their side.　　相手の側から見てみよう
   She **has a point there**.　　彼女の言い分に**一理はある**
   Just making excuses merely **elicits a negative chain reaction**.　　言い訳するだけでは**悪循環を招く**だけだ
3. **Try to identify appropriate positive thinking**　　プラス思考で思索する
   He is **our client**. He must have come here with some health trouble.　　**お客様**である　　@ Customers are always correct.　　お客様は神様である
4. **Replace negative thinking with positive thinking**　　プラス思考に置き換える
   When a delay occurred, I **should've given** them an update and explanation as to the schedule change.　　最新情報を伝える**べきであった**
5. **Select a better emotion and behavior**　　前向きな感情・行動を選択する
   Staff:　　I'm sorry to have kept you waiting so long without any notice. I'll **make it a lesson for myself** next time.　　教訓にする

Case 2

Situation: A staff member who received a bitter scolding from his supervisor finally denied rage over the situation.　　上司に叱責されたスタッフが，最後に激怒を払拭する

Bad example

1. **yielding to** self-hatred　　自己嫌悪に陥る
   I don't believe I adopted such a stupid attitude.
   I am worthless as a medical staff! I really am.
2. Negative thinking **engenders** a negative emotion.　　マイナス思考がマイナス感情を**誘発する**
   I am an experienced professional. I should never have behaved like that.
3. **Putting** the **blame** on another　　他人を**責めはじめる**
   For all that, what an unqualified person he is.　　それにしても
   He just blames me. Why not **give ear to** my excuse?　　耳を傾ける
   He **isn't fit to be a** supervisor at all!　　上司としてまったく**失格**だ

Good example

1. Recognizing a realistic situation.　　現状を把握する
   I can't believe I could make such a stupid mistake!
   No wonder the boss got so upset.　　無理もない
2. Shifting to positive thinking while not denying one's own weaknesses (USA)

自身の全人格を否定せずにプラス思考に移す

I don't want that to **happen again**. 2度とご免だ

But it doesn't mean I'm totally worthless.

It just means that I better be careful to have a more thoughtful attitude next time. ただ〜すればよい

3. Accepting another person with positive thinking (UOA) プラス思考で相手の立場を認める

I didn't like his criticism of me in front of my colleagues.

But **where on earth** does a perfect boss exist? 一体どこに

The way he took it has served **as a good warning to others**. 仲間へのいいみせしめ（scapegoat）として

Quiz

A. What are some stressful situations?
B. What is a popular method for self-control or anger control?
C. What are the three main constructive philosophies of REBT?
D. Describe UOA
E. What does "Unconditional Life Acceptance" mean?
F. What does REBT teach?

Answers

A. Any situation that disturbs everyday activities imposes stress. Most health care involves some stress, and the hospital environment often proves stressful to both patients and medical staff. This is especially true in crisis situations when speed is a factor or when disagreement exists about what should be done in team medicine. Stress is usually higher than ever when working in an emergency room. Sometimes dealing with families can be especially stressful in an emotionally charged situation.
B. Rational Emotive Behavior Therapy (REBT) initiated by Dr. Albert Ellis
C. USA (Unconditional Self Acceptance), UOA (Unconditional Other Acceptance) and ULA (Unconditional Life Acceptance)
D. UOA stands for "Unconditional Other Acceptance," where you never damn other people. You may damn what they do; but you never tell someone they are totally no good, they deserve to die, etc.
E. ULA (Unconditional Life Acceptance) means you don't damn the world. You

accept the fact that things are often very bad, deplorable, sad, but it's not the end of the world. Life goes on.
- **F.** REBT teaches that one can, and should, take responsibility for one's own emotions. That is, one can select one's own emotion or reaction before acting it out, even when the other person, for example a patient, makes unreasonable complaints.

Relevant expressions and additional phrases

1) Cause and effect　原因と結果

An excuse **gives rise to** other's escalating anger. (cause)　　言い訳は怒りを増幅する

Anger **leads to** a negative chain reaction. (elicit)

Stress **results in** depression. (develop)

Hatred **brings about** hatred. (engender)

cf. endanger　危険にさらす

Anger **results** (stems) **from** insult.　　怒りは侮辱から**生じる**

His anger **originated in** the other's insult.　　相手に侮辱**された**ので彼は怒った

His anger **derives from** the insult.　cf. The insult **drove** him to anger.

2) Link words　つなぎ言葉

a) Amplification　増幅

On top of that／Making it even worse　　おまけに（主にnegativeな状況に使用する）

Moreover／Even more／Furthermore／Besides　　それに

b) Concession　譲歩

For all that　それにしても

If you ask me　言わせてもらえば

I don't mean to hurt your feelings, but ~　　悪気で言うのではないですが

3) Emphasis by interrogative and negation　　疑問・否定による強調表現

Where **on earth** can you find a perfect person!　　**一体全体**どこに

Nowhere is there a perfect person!　　完全な人間などどこにもいない

A fool **am I**!　　倒置（inversion）による強調

I should **never ever** have made such a stupid mistake!　　絶対に

4) Singular or plural　　単数か複数か

Idiomatic usage　　慣用表現

He **gave ear to** what I said.　　傾聴した（単数）

He **was all ears to** what I said.　　傾聴した（複数）

He kept **a constant eye** on the child.　　一時も目を放さなかった（単数）

He **took his eyes** off the child for a moment.　　ちょっと目を放した（複数）

He **took a momentary eye** off the child.　　ちょっと目を放した（単数）

They say, "No news **is** good news."　　ニュースは単数扱い

5) Indefinite pronoun　　不定代名詞

Every staff member is well-trained.　　every / each は単数扱い

Everything's OK?　　every の複合形

Each one of the staff members is under training.

All were disappointed.　　人の場合は複数形

All staff members are attending a meeting.

I hope all is going well for you and your family.　　物・事は単数で受ける

All is well that ends well.　　終わりよければすべてよし（諺：シェークスピア）

6) Plural objects　　複数対象

shake hands　　握手する

make friends　　友達になる

change trains　　電車を乗り換える

Exercise I.

Answer the following question in English with 80 words or more. Use as many of the key words and phrases as possible.

Question: What should medical staff take into consideration concerning patient care?

Key words and phrases: the first thing to do（最優先事項は），build rapport, result in, as a result, the last thing we want to do（決してしてはいけないこと），fall short of, in other words（つまり），live up to

Example answerは巻末（付録の前）に掲載

Chapter II.

Emergency
救急医療

1. First Aid　　　　　　　　　　　　　　　　　　　　——応急手当

In an emergency, a citizen (layperson) is usually the first person who recognizes an emergency and tries to help. Ideally, everyone should be trained in **first aid**[*1]. Whoever it may be, he or she needs to **call the local emergency number (dial 9-1-1)** [*2] or notify a nearby **first responder**[*3] for help at the scene of the emergency. Don't hesitate to call. Remember that **EMS** (emergency medical services) **professionals**[*4] would rather respond to a nonemergency than arrive at an emergency too late to help. The first responder may be a firefighter or police officer who is trained to provide a higher level of care. They provide a **critical transition**[*5] until medical professionals arrive. **Paramedics**[*6] are highly specialized professionals who serve as the **field extension**[*7] of the hospital physician and can administer medication, provide advanced airway care and address **abnormal heart rhythms**[*8].

In some cases, individual persons have arrived at scene where they cannot help but do something to rescue a victim even though they are not trained; or are trained, but have little confidence in their skills. Once they dial 9-1-1, a **dispatcher**[*9] answers the call for help and quickly determines what help is needed. The dispatcher works in a **communications center**[*10] for dispatching appropriate professionals according to demands. Their most prominent task is to give the caller instructions over the phone on how best to care for the victim until EMS professionals arrive. Whether citizens are trained or not, most are afraid that what they do may make the situation worse. The worst thing is to do nothing in fear that one might be sued for giving first aid. In order to encourage people to help victims whose lives may be endangered, most states have enacted "**Good Samaritan" laws**[*11] to give legal protection to citizens and medical professionals. These laws are prepared for those who act in good faith to provide emergency assistance to ill or injured persons at the scene of an emergency. These laws may not apply in cases when a rescuer's response is **grossly**[*12] or **willfully negligent**[*13], or when he doesn't ask a conscious victim for **permission**[*14] before giving care.

Notes: *1 第一救護（応急手当），*2 救急要請電話番号（米国では救急・火災ともに911，参考1参照），*3 救急医療士（消防・警察局に所属し，主に一次救命処置を行うtechnician, EMT），*4 救急医療士，*5 救急医療士から特別救急医療士までの救急処置移行期間，*6 特別救急医療士（二次救命処置と呼ばれる気管内挿管：endotracheal intubation，投薬，除細動等の資格を有する隊員），*7 野外病院，*8 不整脈：arrhythmia，*9 指令員，*10 救急災害情報センター，*11 Reference 参照，*12 まったくでたらめに，*13 未必の故意で（cf: professional negligence：職務怠慢，homicide by negligence：障害致死），*14 i.e. informed consent：納得診療

Dialogue

Situation :

A driver got out of the car because she had a flat tire. Another car couldn't stop in time and hit her. The victim was thrown on the road. The driver of the car hesitated to stop, but drove off in a flurry (hit-and-run). The following car stopped. The driver quickly approached the victim and dialed 9-1-1 using his cellular phone. Following, a **dispatcher**, Robert, promptly gives him instructions about first aid.

タイヤがパンクしたので女性ドライバーが車から降りる。後続の車が停止しようとしたが，間に合わず彼女を撥ねた。女性は道路に飛ばされた。加害者は引き返そうとは思いながらも慌てて逃走した。次の車が停止した。ドライバーは彼女にかけ寄り，携帯電話で緊急要請の911番に電話した。ロバートという**司令員**が迅速に彼に応急手当の指示を与える。

Caller: Traffic accident! The victim is a middle-aged woman. Seems to be a severe head wound. I'm calling from Bear Valley.

Robert: I'm Robert Smith. Does she respond to you?

Caller: No. She is conscious but restless. Can't speak. Maybe injured in the back of her head. I see a lot of blood spreading on the road.

Robert: Is she lying on her back?

Chapter II. Emergency 27

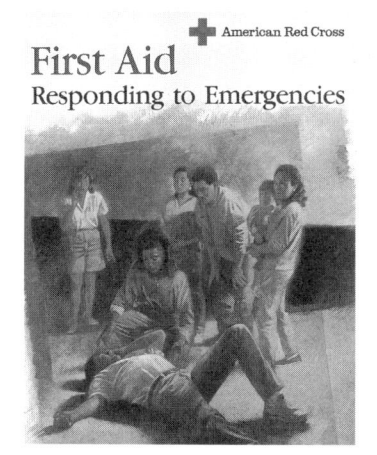

Fig. 1 A Textbook edited by the American Red Cross who issues the first aid course completion certificate for those who pass the examination (See Reference 1).
米国赤十字社で編集された応急手当認定試験用の教科書（文献1参照）

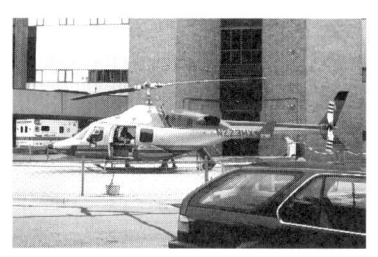

Fig. 2 A helicopter standing by the ER area which responds to emergencies with in a 150 mile radius.
救急医療室脇に待機しているヘリコプターは，半径240km範囲を受け持つ。

Caller: Yes. So I can't see the injured area clearly. Also, her hair hides the wound. What should I do?

Robert: Are you trained in first aid?

Caller: **Yes and No**. I have a **CPR certificate (Fig. 1)**, but I am not sure what to do in this case.　　あいまいな返事（補足1参照）／心肺蘇生術講習の終了認定書

Robert: Try to move her head and neck as little as possible. She might have injuries there. If you have a handkerchief, fold it with the clean side out. Place it over the wound and apply mild pressure with your hand holding the dressing. If you feel a depression or bone fragments, don't put direct pressure on the wound. Is there any bystander?

Caller: Yes. Here comes a car.

Robert: I've asked **UWH** (University of Wisconsin Hospital) to dispatch a helicopter. It will soon be ready to fly. Tell me the precise position (**Fig. 2**).
ウィスコンシン大学病院

Caller: (to a male driver) Is your car equipped with a car navigator? I need our exact

	location.
Robert:	Don't hang up the phone until I hang up.
Caller:	He tells me, Route 130 and 10 miles up or north of the intersection point with Highway 14.
Robert:	On Route 130, 10 miles north of Highway 14. I got it. It's 40 miles northwest of the hospital. Wait about 20 minutes. Is there any landmark building?
Caller:	No, I see only silos about two miles apart. We are **right in a sea of fields**. 畑の大海原のど真ん中
Robert:	Is the road wide enough for the helicopter to land, with no hindrances like **utility poles**?　電信柱のような障害物
Caller:	It's wide and clear enough.
Robert:	Now, the helicopter just left. The road has been closed. The police are searching for the assaulter's car, a blue station wagon heading north, right?
Caller:	Yes, but I missed the license number. Oh, her breathing is becoming faster and face looks pale.
Robert:	Her heart is **compensating**. With the loss of blood, the heart is beating faster to meet the body's demands for oxygen. More blood is reserved for the vital organs reducing amount for less important tissue, like the skin. The lungs also breathe faster for needed oxygen. So she looks pale and cold even with rapid breathing. Blood loss increases with the heart beat. Is she still bleeding? 代償行動をしている（Domino effect 参照）
Caller:	**I had better call** it oozing from the handkerchief rather than bleeding. 〜と言ったほうがよい The small handkerchief of mine couldn't absorb all the blood. It is like I applied pressure directly with my bare hand. Oh, someone has taken off his T-shirt trying to secure the dressing with it. That will help.
Robert:	Even if the bleeding stops, don't remove the blood-soaked dressing, or the clot may tear away with it. Police cars will arrive there soon.
Caller:	Oh, no! She vomited.
Robert:	Please monitor her airway and breathing.
Caller:	She is breathing very rapidly and wheezing, and has become quite pale and drowsy. In other words she's almost lost consciousness.
Robert:	Keep calm. It's usually the case in shock. Do you know **"in-line stabilization?"**　中心線安定化（参考2参照）

Chapter II. Emergency

Caller: Yes, I'm also suspecting the possibility of neck injuries.

Robert: Listen. Make sure to minimize the movement of her head and neck. Ask someone to help roll her gently onto her side while you **keep the head and spine in as straight a line as possible**.　"中心線安定化"の指示

Treat her body as a whole unit. Rest her chin on her bent arm facing your side. If you know the **Coma position**, try to decline the spine line to clear any **vomit**. 昏睡位（半伏臥位）（参考3参照）／吐瀉物

Caller: Yes, I understand. We'll roll her a little bit forward to raise her hip higher than her head.

Robert: OK? ------ Good. Well done! Do you hear sirens? It's about time for either police officers or flight paramedics to arrive.

Caller: I can hear a siren. And, it sounds like a helicopter in the distance. Do you think she will be saved?

Robert: It depends on the brain damage. In general, the chance for survival is not high for victims who go into shock from a mild case of the **Domino effect**.　ドミノ効果（参考4参照）

Don't be discouraged even if she doesn't make it. You should feel assured that you have done everything you could to help. Wisconsin protects you under the **Good Samaritan laws**, whatever the result.　よきサマリア人法（Exercise 2参照）

That's why I assisted you in helping her. You are to be commended for your brave effort. You faithfully followed my directions and continued to care for her in the life-threatening condition until EMS personnel could arrive. My phone is linked with the medical professionals and police officers. They have been listening to my call to you and known how things are going.

Notes

1. **A local emergency number** is prepared for the ambulance in a **jurisdiction office**. 救急要請電話番号は救急車の派遣を**管轄署**に依頼するためにある。＠番号は国内共通であるが，管轄範囲が地域分担となるので local number と呼ばれる。

2. **In-line stabilization** is a maneuver, when spinal injuries are suspected, for minimizing movement of the head and neck keeping the spinal column as natural as possible.

3. The **Coma position** is assumed so an unconscious victim will have a free airpas-

sage and the tongue does not fall backwards to block it. Also, you can expel **vomit** in case there is any.　吐瀉物

4 The **Domino effect** is the **compensation** of the heart to quickly adjust circulation of the blood by giving priority to the vital organs. The amount of blood flow to the less important tissues decreases by contracting the blood vessels in the arms, legs and skin. The brain, in turn, sends a signal to supply blood to these minor parts according to their minimal necessity and the heart tries to balance the blood flow with the vital organs. The body's continuous attempt to compensate for blood loss will cause **decompensation** for the heart which may result in death.　代償効果／（心臓の）代償不全

Quiz

A. Why are Good Samaritan laws enacted in many states in America?
B. Who are usually the first responders?
C. What is the prominent assignment of a dispatcher?
D. What do A, B and C stand for in the first check of a victim?
E. Why should one not remove a blood-soaked pad from a wound when trying to control bleeding?

Answers

A. Good Samaritan laws are enacted to give legal protection to citizens and medical professionals in order to encourage people to help victims whose lives may be endangered.
B. They may be firefighters, police officers, industrial safety officers, or whoever are trained to provide a higher level of care.
C. The dispatcher gives a caller instructions about how to help until EMS personnel arrive.
D. They stand for Airway, Breathing and Circulation.
E. When bleeding stops, platelets start to form a clot for covering the area and controlling bleeding. If the dressing is removed, part or all of the clot may be torn away with it.

2. Cardiac Arrest　　　　　　　　　　　　——心停止

CPR (Cardiopulmonary resuscitation) *1 is an emergency lifesaving procedure that combines **rescue breathing***2 (which provides oxygen to the victim's lungs) and **chest compression***3 (which keeps the victim's heart circulating oxygenated blood) to restart the heart and lungs. Chest compression is performed only when the heartbeat has stopped. Unnecessary chest compression causes harm to the victim. Remember that **compression alone will not sustain the life of a victim***4 since the body tissue needs oxygen-rich blood. Given together, breathing and chest compressions (CPR), can artificially take over the function of the lungs and heart. When cardiac arrest occurs, breathing ceases before long. Permanent damage to the brain can occur if blood flow is not restored within four to six minutes. This **irreversible***5 damage to brain cells is known as **biological death***6. CPR can be lifesaving, but it is best performed by those who have CPR training. It is also important to know that CPR techniques vary slightly depending on the age or size of the victim. Be sure also that even under the best of conditions, **CPR only generates about one third of the normal blood flow to the brain***7. This is why it is important to call EMS personnel immediately. They can provide **advanced life support (ALS)** *8 wherever they are called. Defibrillation is the key to helping victims survive cardiac arrest. A **defibrillator***9 is a device which sends an electric shock through the victim's chest to resume a **functional heartbeat***10. An easy-to-use automatic one has recently been used widely. When speed is critical, as in the case of cardiac arrest an untrained person should shout for help and immediately make an emergency call. When a person who has recently trained in CPR is confronted with a real cardiac arrest situation, he or she will face a dilemma, which to do first ----- she call the EMS personnel or perform CPR, or vice versa? If one feels confident about their skill, CPR should be the first option. However, you should not do it more than **4 cycles***11. If no one still responds to your shouts, go to the nearest phone, leaving the victim behind, and come back quickly to resume CPR.

Notes: *1 心肺蘇生術, *2 人工呼吸, *3 心臓マッサージ, *4 心臓マッサージだけでは被害者の生命を維持できない, *5 回復不能の, *6 生物学死, *7 CPRだけでは正常時の1／3の血流しか脳に行かない, *8 二次救命処置, *9 除細動器, *10 自発拍動, *11 15回心臓マッサージ＋2回吸気吹き込みを1回動作としたときの4反復（約1分）

Dialogue

Situation :

Kathy, a high school student, finds her father collapsed on the floor. She has learned CPR at school but is uncertain about how to actually give it. Receiving no response to " Are you OK?," she quickly runs to her father's side. He first makes noises but soon becomes silent. She shouts for help from her mother watering flowers in the garden. Kathy is so stunned and upset that she forgets the basic rule for minimally-trained persons in CPR like her, "Shout for help and call the local emergency number as soon as possible."

In the following dialogue, the caller's talking to a dispatcher over the phone is given in parentheses, < >, and the recited words are put in quotation marks.

高校生のキャシーは父が床に倒れるのをみる。高校でCPRについて習ってはいるが，実際に行うとなると自信がない。父に"大丈夫"と呼びかけたが返事がないので急いでかけ寄る。父は大きな呼吸音をたてていたが，やがて静かになった。庭で花に水をやっていた母に大声で助けを求める。あまりの驚きと動転で，彼女のようなCPR未熟者に対する鉄則，"助けを求めた後にすぐに救急要請電話をすること"を忘れてしまった。

下記の会話で，司令員との電話での会話を鍵括弧< >，指令を復唱する部分をイタリック体で記して引用符" "で囲む。

Mother: Have you dialed 9-1-1? Is he breathing? Check the pulse.

Kathy: I haven't called yet. He is breathing, but when I shouted to him, he just made noises.

Mother: Make a phone call quickly! Meanwhile, I will do CPR.

Kathy: < No,---- no time to take a pulse. ---- Mom says "No pulse." > Mom, not on the wrist (radial artery). He says "grab both sides of his Adam's apple (for carotid pulse) firmly with your fingers and thumb."

< Mom says, "All the same." ---- Even worse, " Fainting in breathing." > Mom, don't straddle his stomach. **Kneel beside his chest.** Don't push on the left, but on the sternum, breastbone. Keep your fingers off the chest, or you'll break his ribs. I didn't know you're really a greenhorn! You don't know the first thing about CPR, indeed! **Let me do it for you.** You take the phone. The dispatcher will instruct us what to do.　　父の胸脇に跪く／役割を交換した

Chapter II. Emergency 33

Mom:	方がよい ＜Yes, she is rechecking his pulse, ---- Now, she's tilting his head and lifting his chin.＞ ＜Yes, I'll repeat your instructions.＞ Kathy, "*Over the lower half of the sternum. Two finger-widths above the lowest notch.*" Kathy, he says he can hear you. Keep speaking with a loud voice.
Kathy:	I know the hand position. How many pushes and breaths?
Mom:	He says, "15 compressions and 2 breaths, and count aloud as you push down." "It helps you pace yourself, and also he can hear you counting." Kathy, follow my instructions quickly.
Kathy:	OK, Mom. "One, two, three,--- "
Mom:	He says it's too fast. Like this, one and two and three and--- . **Put the word "and" as you release the pressure**.　手を緩めるとき "の" の字を入れなさい。1 の 2 の 3 の 4 の......ように ＜Yes, she should place her other hand directly on top of the first hand. ---- Yes, I'll repeat you.＞ "*Don't bend your arms. Lock your elbows.*" "**Lean your shoulders over your hands**, *and firmly press down about 2 inches into his chest.*" "*Move in a smooth and rhythmic manner with no pause between compressions.*"　手と肩の位置が直角になるまで前のめりになって
Kathy:	When shall I recheck the pulse?
Mom:	"*After 4 cycles of compression and breaths.*" "*One cycle takes about 1 minute.*" "*Check the pulse within 5 minutes.*"　1 サイクルはリード文注釈参照
Kathy:	OK. Continue talking to him for further details.
Mom:	"*If there's still no pulse, give him two full breaths and continue* **CPR**." "*Recheck* **chin up / head down**." Kathy, has it already been one minute? 頭部後屈
Kathy:	No pulse, now. Every minute, or each cycle for the next time, too?
Mom:	"*Every few minutes from the next time.*" OK?
Kathy:	Mom, Dad is making a noise! He's gasping for air, wheezing!
Mom:	He says, stop CPR and check the pulse.
Kathy:	We did it! He opened his eyes!

Quiz

A. Why is it necessary to check the airway first during a primary survey of an unconscious victim?

B. Why should the head be tilted back and the chain lifted up for an unconscious victim?

C. Why is it necessary to check the carotid pulse when the victim is unconscious?

D. When do you start and not start CPR?

E. Why are chest compression and rescuer breathing both necessary for CPR?

F. Why do you need to call for a professional's help, and why apply CPR as quickly as possible?

Answers

A. To make sure that the victim's airway is not blocked by the tongue falling into the back of the throat or by a foreign body.

B. To move the tongue away from the back of the throat, allowing air to enter the lungs.

C. In a coma state, blood flow to the extremities is much less than to the vital organs like the brain, so the radial pulse is very weak.

D. When a victim is breathing, but has no heart beat. Unneeded chest compression may cause the heart to stop beating.

E. The heart transports blood to the organs, but the organs need oxygen.

F. Without CPR, the brain begins to die within four to six minutes. However, CPR only generates about one third of the normal blood flow to the brain.

3. Respiratory Arrest ——呼吸停止

Respiratory arrest is the condition in which breathing stops. It occurs from direct causes or results from respiratory distress such as asthma, **hyperventilation**[1] and **anaphylactic shock**[2]. Direct causes include illness, injury and an obstructed airway. Without oxygen for a few minutes, the heart muscle stops functioning, causing other body systems to fail. **Rescue breathing**[3] is given to victims who are not breathing but still have a pulse. **Airway obstruction**[4], either anatomical or mechanical, is the most common cause of respiratory emergency. Anatomical obstruction may result from injury to the neck or anaphylactic shock which can progress into laryngeal and **bronchial edema**[5] causing respiratory arrest. When victims become unconscious, their muscles, especially the tongue, become relaxed being deprived of oxygen. The maneuver of tilting the head back and the jaw forward not only opens the airway by moving the tongue away from the back of the throat, but also moves the soft tissue (**epiglottis***6) flap from the opening of the **trachea**.*7 The epiglottis is a special soft tissue that covers the airway (laryngeal opening) when swallowing to prevent food and liquid from entering the lungs. On the other hand, **mechanical airway obstruction or choking***8 occurs if someone tries to swallow large pieces of poorly chewed food. In this case, victims are usually quite **agitated***9, he or she **becomes congested***10 in the face, and may tear at the collar or clutch the throat. In addition to CPR, it is beneficial for anyone to know how to perform abdominal thrusts or **Heimlick maneuver***11. One stands behind the victim and quickly and forcefully applies pressure upward against the **diaphragm***12 just below the ribs. This simulates a cough, forcing air trapped in the lungs to push the **aspirated object***13 out of the airway.

Notes: *1 呼吸亢進, *2 過敏症 i.e. anapyhlaxis, *3 救命呼吸法（呼気吹き込み法：expired air resuscitation）cf. spontaneous respiration:（回復後の）自発呼吸, *4 気道閉塞（解剖学的, 機械的）, *5 喉頭・気管支浮腫, *6 喉頭蓋, *7 気管, *8 気道障害（窒息）, *9 動揺する, *10 充血する, *11 ハイムリック手法, *12 横隔膜（発音に注意）, *13 誤嚥物 cf. vomit（吐瀉物）

Dialogue

Situation :

When a father tries to swallow a big piece of meat, it gets lodged in his throat. His son shouts for help from his mother in the kitchen. The mother comes and stands behind the father to give him abdominal thrusts, but fails. The situation worsens to respiratory arrest. The son calls 9-1-1, and repeats aloud the instructions made by a dispatcher to his mother. *Here, his recited words are put in quotation marks.*

父が大きな肉の塊を飲み込もうとして，咽を詰まらせてしまった。息子は大きな声でキッチンにいた母に助けを求める。母は父の背中側に立ちハイムリック手法を行う。状況は悪化し呼吸停止となる。息子は911に電話をして司令員の指示を母に伝達する。

注：ここでは，息子の指示反復を引用符" "で囲む

Son: Dad can't speak, Mom. His face is congested.   充血している

Mom:	Wait honey. I'll sweep it out now.
Son:	No, not now!
Mom:	Ouch. He bit my finger severely.
Son:	He's turning pale. You might have pushed the obstruction deeper into his throat.
Mom:	Oh, no. He's gone unconscious. Call emergency quickly.
Son:	You should've called first!
Mom:	**Don't cry over split milk!**　　いまさら何よ
Son:	The dispatcher says, "Lower him to the floor on his back. And give him two full breaths." Don't forget, Mom, the head- tilt / chin-lift!
Mom:	I know it well. Don't worry.
Son:	No, don't do CPR. He just says, "Give two full breaths and recheck the object." He (the dispatcher) says he can hear you, shouting at me each time.
Mom:	The meat is still lodged in his throat.
Son:	"*Give 6 to 10 **abdominal thrusts**.*"　　お腹をしゃくりあげる
Mom:	I've done it many times, as you can see.
Son:	"*He is unconscious, so the **throat muscle will relax enough to allow air to pass the object**.*" Do as he says, OK? .　　のどの筋肉が緩んで息がのどを通る
Mom:	It still won't come out. What's next?
Son:	"*After the thrusts, give two full breaths.*" "*And, try the finger sweep again.*" 指払い（他方の指で口を固定し，利き手の人差し指で行う。幼児には使用しない）
Mom:	I did! I swept it out! ------ Wait. He isn't breathing.
Son:	How about the pulse? OK? You should start rescue breathing.
Mom.	How is it different from CPR?
Son:	"*Kneel next to his chin and pinch his nose.*"　　顎のそばに跪き，鼻をつまむ He warns you. "*Be confident and dad will restart breathing on his own for sure.*" "*Breathe in slowly and see if his chest rises.*"
Mom:	I don't think my breaths will go in.
Son:	"*Tilt his head back far enough .*" "*Don't blow too fast and give one breath every five seconds.*" "*Each breath should last one to one and a half seconds, with a pause in-between to let the air flow back out.*" "*Check the pulse after every 12 breaths.*"
Mom:	You're speaking too fast!

Son: "*Count aloud to ensure a pause, like this-one one-thousand*, two one-thousand, three one-thousand, put the word "one-thousand", then take a breath yourself before breathing in.*" 間隔を確認するので大きな声で数えなさい。一価千分の一，二価千分の一，三価千分の一と言うように，"千分の一" *の言葉を追加してから息を吸い込み，それから息を吹き込みなさい。

    *正式には，一価千分の一は one and one thousandth, 一価千分の二は one and two thousandths と読む（分子が複数ならば分母も複数となる）。

Mom: I hear a siren wailing toward us.

Son: Continue the breathing until they take over for you.

Quiz

    A. Why do you need to pause between each rescue breath?
    B. Why can't rescue breathing alone sustain the life of anyone without a pulse?
    C. Why is anaphylactic shock a life-threatening emergency?
    D. How and when do food and other objects get stuck in the trachea?
    E. How can abdominal thrusts expel choking objects?
    F. Why do abdominal thrusts become more effective if a victim becomes unconscious?
    G. When a foreign body becomes lodged in the opening of the trachea, how does the victim behave?
    H. What should you do before you apply the Heimlic maneuver?
    I. Why should you not insert fingers in an effort to retrieve an obstructed object for a victim who is quite agitated?
    J. If foreign material is visible in the mouth of an unconscious adult victim, how do you retrieve the material?

Answers

    A. In order to let the air flow back out.
    B. Without a working heart, oxygen can not be delivered to body tissues.
    C. Because swollen tissues of the mouth and throat impairs breathing.
    D. When one eats, the epiglottis functions to cover the opening of the trachea so that food and liquid cannot enter the lungs. When a person tries to breathe and swallow at the same time, especially if eating a bigger object than is readily chewable, choking can occur.
    E. It simulates a cough, forcing air trapped in the lungs to push the aspirated object out of the airway.

F. The victim's throat muscle relaxes enough to allow air to pass the object.

G. A victim usually becomes quite agitated, the face becomes congested, and he may tear at his collar or clutch his throat.

H. Ask the victim if he can speak; if he does not answer, tell him what you are about to do.

I. Severe bite can occur, and the obstructing material can be forced further into the throat during the struggle.

J. Grasp the victim's tongue and lower the jaw. Insert the index finger of the other hand to the base of the tongue, and sweep it forward to clear the obstruction.

4. Hospital emergency procedures (anaphylaxisis)
——病院救急医療（過敏症）

Severe allergic reaction to poison is rare. But when it does occur, it is truly a life-threatening medical emergency. The reaction in this case is called **anaphylaxis**[*1], a form of shock. It can be caused by an insect bite or sting, or by contact with drugs, medications or chemicals. One of the most common medical emergencies in hospitals is a reaction to **contrast media**[*2]. As opposed to anaphylaxis that usually occurs within seconds or minutes after contact with an allergen, an adverse reaction to **iodinated contrast media**[*3] may not occur for up to 30 minutes in some cases. **On top of that**[*4], even a patient who has been given contrast media without an adverse reaction is **not necessarily free of**[*5] having a reaction with a second injection. Most reactions occur immediately following an injection, as a direct response to it, turning the skin red with hives, itching and / or rash. In a *mild* case, a reaction may appear as a cough, **dizziness**[*6], itching or **pruritus**[*7], nasal **stuffiness**[*8], headache, shaking, minimal rash or **hives**[*9] and mild facial swelling. *Moderate* reactions include **tachycardia**[*10] or **bradycardia**[*11], moderate or severe **urticaria**[*12], **dyspnea**[*13], mild **laryngeal edema**[*14], hypertension and hypotension, and bronchial spasms accompanied by **wheezing**[*15]. A *severe* reaction can quickly develop into a life threatening condition such as respiratory or cardiac arrest. It may also include moderate to severe laryngeal edema, **convulsions**[*16], **contraction**[*17], **profound or protracted hypotension**[*18], **clinically manifest arrhythmia**[*19] and / or cardio-pulmonary arrest.

Before the procedure of giving contrast media, you as a health provider should review the patient's history asking yourself the following questions: 1) Is he/she diabetic? 2)

What medication is he / she taking?   3) Could that medication **react adversely to**[20] an IV contrast injection?   4) Should the medication be suspended for 48 hours before or after the contrast injection?   Make sure you are alert to the possibility of a reaction and that you are prepared should one occur.

Notes: *1 過敏症，*2 造影剤，*3 ヨード系造影剤，*4 おまけに，*5 必ずしも～とはかぎらない，*6 めまい，*7 痒み，*8 鼻づまり，*9 湿疹，*10 頻拍，*11 遅脈，*12 蕁麻疹，*13 呼吸困難，*14 喉頭浮腫，*15 呼気性ぜん鳴（笛音）: i.e. expiratory w.，*16 痙攣，*17 攣縮，*18 低いまま長引く血圧降下，*19 臨床的に明白な不整脈，*20 禁忌である

@ degree of severity 重篤度（mild: 軽度の，moderate: 中程度の，severe: 重篤な）

Dialogue

A junior RN (JRN) notices a patient starts developing a breathing problem while she is staying with him following an intravenous injection of contrast media. Before long, she notices his condition turning worse, and runs next door to get help from a senior RN (SRN). The radiologist in charge of the patient (R) arrives at the scene for immediate care. He has the nurse call **cor-o**[1] and asks for the **crash cart**, but finally the patient is transferred to the emergency unit.

新人看護師（JRN）が造影剤の静脈注射の後しばらく患者の様子をみていたが，患者の呼吸の様子がおかしいのに気づく。容態が急変したので隣の部屋にいた先輩看護師（SRN）の助けを求めにかけていく。担当の放射線科医（R）は**救急室（コー・オー）**[1]に**救急カート**を求めるが，最終的に患者は救急室に運ばれる。

JRN: My patient is complaining of nausea and has vomited after severe coughing. He seems to be having an adverse reaction to the contrast media.

SRN: Oh no. We must report this to the radiologist immediately. Have you checked the vital signs?

JRN: I was so rushed that I wasn't able to. I was busy clearing vomit from his mouth and **keeping** his **airway** open. It was impossible for me alone to keep him in a **head down and chin up position**. He is restless.
嘔吐物の除去と気道確保で精一杯，自分ひとりでは頭部後屈／下顎挙上の位置を保つのは不可能

SRN: Let's check the signs before the doctor comes. I can see urticaria (hives) on

	his arms. Skin color is pale. What is his BP?
JRN:	70 over 50.
SRN:	He's breathing rapidly. What is the respiratory rate?
JRN:	Shallow and rapid respiration...40 per minute.
SRN:	The symptoms of hypotension and tachypnea may indicate more than a **mild case** of anaphylactic shock. Fold the blanket so that we can elevate his legs. Elevate them higher, please, until they are clearly above the level of the heart, and the blood in the legs is able to reach the brain. Like that. I'll bring an O₂ set. Give him **O$_2$ via the nose mask**.　ベンマスクによる酸素吸入をしなさい
JRN:	He's experiencing tachycardia! His pulse rate is 100 and irregular.
	Radiologist (R) runs into the room.　放射線科医が駆け込んでくる。
R:	Let me know his vital signs. Give me one milliliter of diluted epinephrine please. After I inject it, start an IV (intravenous) saline infusion. Can you hear the expiratory wheezing? His breathing has turned to **forced respiration**. 呼吸が**努力呼吸**に変わった
SRN:	We have **endotracheal intubation** equipment here in this room. 気管内挿管の器具がこの部屋に備えてある
R:	We cannot apply the intubation technique on a conscious patient because **gag reflex** may occur. It could cause not only tracheal injury, but also **laryngospasms**.　気管内挿管を行うと**上気道反射**を起こすかもしれない／気管の損傷のほかに**喉頭痙攣**を招く
JRN:	His level of consciousness is worsening. He's not responding to me well.
R:	Has his BP risen?
JRN:	No, not yet. And I can still hear irregular **spurts of blood flow**. まだ不規則な**血流音**がしている
R:	Profound hypotension and clinical manifest arrhythmia are signs of an emergency case. Call cor-o and ask for the crash cart. He needs prolonged airway and circulatory management immediately. He may have severe **laryngeal edema** associated with **tachyarrhythmia**.　頻拍性不整脈を伴った重度の喉頭浮腫が起こるおそれがある
SRN:	We thought you would bring him back to his room soon. We've prepared most of the emergency medications and equipment in his room.
R:	His condition declined much faster than I imagined it would. Such a serious

case is very rare. We are happy to know his condition is stable now. **EMS personnel** are continuing to monitor his condition **around the clock**. I'm thinking I should have called them earlier, since they are the appropriate professionals for handling such a situation. They performed a **tracheostomy**, abandoning intubation **on the verge of** cardio-pulmonary arrest. I will **go tell** his wife that there will be no more problems.

救急医療士が**24時間体制**で彼の容態を監視すると言った／心肺停止に瀕していたので気管内挿管を諦めて**気管切開術**を行った／彼の妻のもとに行って，もう安心と**告げてくる**

In the room after returning from the emergency unit. 　　救急医療室から戻って

JRN: Wow! I was surprised and **fell to pieces**. 　　びっくりして**あがってしまった**

SRN: So did I. In my long career, I've never had such a severe case.

R: To tell the truth, **neither have** I. Fatalities from an allergic reaction to intravenous injection of contrast media is said to be **one out of a hundred thousand** cases. You both **deserve credit for** your heroic efforts in helping me correctly. 　　実は私も**初めての経験**／死に至るケースは**10万回に1回**と言われている／果敢に私の指示に従った2人の努力は**表彰**ものである

SRT: I think we are all familiar with CPR and the Heimlich maneuver. But how many of us have ever had to perform these procedures? Today's case teaches us we need to be familiar with all of the emergency techniques used in such situations since one does not usually know when an emergency might suddenly occur.

JRN: We've learned one must always examine a patient closely and **discharge the patient** only after a physician has assessed the condition. In this case, symptoms appeared right away and the patient's condition worsened abruptly.
医師の確認の後に**患者を帰宅させる**

SRT: Yes, that's true. After an exam, we know we must double check to make sure the patient is really OK, and **not just assume he / she is OK**. Many patients are **NPO** prior to an exam. Such patients feel anxiety during the exam and then may become **light-headed and pass out** after the exam due to collapse and / or side effects. 　　検査後は，**大丈夫だろうとの推測**でなく，確認をしなければならない。多くの患者は検査前に**絶食**をして，検査中は不安を感じ，検査後に副作用とは別に脱力感から**気が遠くなり気絶する**ことがある

JRT: My colleague told me, the other day, she found her patient sitting in a chair out-

side the department **holding his head while resting from dizziness**.
目まいがして，頭を抱えて座り込んでいる

Note: ＊1 救急室（coronary care unit）の略（救急医療の対象が主に心疾患であるため）

Quiz

A. What are five mild reactions that might occur after injection of an iodinated contrast media?
B. What are five symptoms that might occur as moderate reactions?
C. What are five symptoms that might occur as severe reactions?
D. Why should the patient not be left unattended until the x-ray examination is completed?
E. Why should you be alert even with patients who have been given contrast media without any problems?
F. In what condition do you think epinephrine is used in an emergency case?
G. Why is syncope, otherwise known as fainting, a common occurrence before an exam?
H. What is the immediate procedure you should under take for a fainted patient? Why?

Answers

A. 1) Erythema (redness)　2) Minimum rash or hives　3) Itching or pruritus　4) Cough　5) Dizziness
B. 1) Tachycardia or bradycardia　2) Moderate or severe urticaria　3) Dyspnea　4) Mild laryngeal edema　5) Hypertension or hypotension
C. 1) Laryngeal edema　2) convulsions　3) profound or protracted hypotension　4) Clinical manifest arrhythmias　5) Cardio-pulmonary arrest
D. Because any reaction may not become apparent up to 30 minutes after an injection.
E. They are not necessary free of having a reaction with a second injection.
F. When a patient shows tachycardia.
G. Many patients are NPO for several hours, or may be experiencing feelings of anxiety prior to a procedure.
H. The immediate response would be to place the patient in a dorsal recumbent position with the feet elevated above the level of the heart. Fainting occurs when the blood pressure is too low to supply the brain with oxygen, so this position helps

increase blood flow back to the brain.

Relative expressions and additional phrases

1) Idiomatic expressions of negation　　否定を表す慣用表現

① A person who doesn't have an adverse reaction is **not necessarily free of** having a reaction with a second injection.　（過去の検査で副作用がなかったからといって）今度もないとは**言いきれない**

② **Who knows** (=No one knows) if the patient will be free from a reaction this time?　修辞疑問：疑問文の形で強い否定

③ I **know better than to** overlook even mild reactions.　見逃す**ほど愚かではない**

④ CPR only generates about one third of normal blood flow to the brain.

⑤ CPR carried out at an accident site is **no where near** the procedures often undertaken in an emergency room.　現地で行われるCPRはERでの処置に**足元にも及ばない**

⑥ Compression alone would not sustain the life of the victim.

⑦ Chest compression is **anything but** a perfect alternative maneuver.　胸骨圧迫は**決して**完全な（自発呼吸の）代償行為**ではない**

2) Idiomatic expressions of bare infinitive　　原形不定詞の慣用表現

① **I had better call** it oozing from handkerchiefs rather than bleeding.　出血というよりハンカチから血が滲み出ていると**言ったほうがよい**。

② It would be **better called** oozing from handkerchiefs than bleeding.

③ I didn't know you're really a greenhorn! (= You don't know the first thing about CPR, indeed!)　I **would rather take** it for you.　ずぶの素人とは知らなかった（いろはの"い"の字も知らないとは）。私が代わってCPRをする**ほうがまし**。

④ Call emergency quickly.　You'd **better dial** 911 right now.　　（提案より命令）

3) Link words (amplification)　　つなぎ言葉（増幅）

1) **On top of that**, even a patient who has been given contrast media without an adverse reaction is **not necessarily free of** having a reaction with a second injection.　おまけに，過去の検査で副作用がなかったからといって

2) **Make it even worse (More over, Even more , Furthermore)**, an adverse reaction to iodinated contrast media may not occur for up to 30 minutes in some cases.　おまけに，ヨード系造影剤による副作用は，場合によっては30分経つまで現れない。

4) Compound medical words　合成医学用語

1. Prefix　接頭語

a, ar は否定または欠乏で，dys は困難，hyper は上で hypo は下，tachy は急速で brady は遅い

2. Suffix　接尾語

phasia は言語の異常，pnea は呼吸，cardia は心臓，ia は病的状態，tension は圧力

1 と 2 を組み合わせると，

aphasia：失語症，dysphasia：発声困難，hypertension：高血圧，hypotension：低血圧，urticaria (urticant 蕁麻疹発生の + ia)：蕁麻疹，arrhythmia (ar + rhythm律動 + ia)：不整脈，apnea：無呼吸，dyspnea：呼吸困難，tachycardia：頻拍，tachypnea：頻呼吸，bradycardia：徐脈，bradypnea：（緩）徐呼吸

5) Taking vital signs　バイタルサインを調べる

Vital signs are used for assessment of a patient's health condition that involve the measurement of: 1) temperature, 2) pulse rate, 3) respiratory rate and 4) blood pressure.

1. Temperature helps accurately measure the body's basic metabolic state. Normal **oral** temperatures[*1] vary from 98.2 degrees Fahrenheit to 99.6 degrees Fahrenheit or 36.6 degrees to 37.6 degrees Celsius. **Rectal** temperatures[*2] range from 0.5 to 1.0 degree higher than oral temperatures, while **axillary** temperatures[*3] range from 0.5 to 1.0 degree lower.

2. **Pulse**[*4] is an easy and effective way to measure **heart rate**[*5]. Average normal pulse rates in adults vary between 60 and 100 beats per minute. When the heart beats are more than or less than this range, they are called Tachycardia or Bradycardia. Common pulse points are the temporal, carotid, apical, radial, femoral and pedal. The most common site for palpitation of the pulse is the radial artery at the base of either thumb.

3. Tachypnea is defined as a **respiratory rate** [*6] faster than the normal level ranging from 14 to 20 respirations per minute. When the rate is slower than the normal average level, it is called bradypnea.

4. Blood pressure (BP) is higher when the heart contracts and blood enters into the arteries, and is called the **systolic blood pressure**[*7]. On the other hand, the **diastolic BP**[*8] is measured at the **diastolic level**[*9] between each heart beat. The two BP readings are recorded such as 130 / 80 and are read 130 over 80. Hypertension

or hypotension is defined as blood pressure that is higher or lower than the average depending on age.

Notes: ＊1 口腔内検温，＊2 直腸検温，＊3 腋窩検温，＊4 心拍，＊5 脈拍数，＊6 呼吸数，＊7 収縮期血圧（最高血圧），＊8 拡張期血圧（最低血圧），＊9 最低血圧レベル

Exercise II.

II-1. Answer the following question in English with 80 words or more.
Title: Why should medical staff learn first aid skills?

II-2. Translate the following sentence into Japanese.

　Good Samaritan laws are based on the well-known parable in the Bible, where the man who, during a journey, aided an injured stranger on the side of the road. These are state laws enacted to give legal protection (legal immunity) to citizens and medical professionals. Anyone should understand how their state laws protect them. When persons respond to an emergency and act as a reasonable and prudent rescuer, Good Samaritan laws apply to them regardless of the outcome. However, rescuers should not exceed the scope of their training. They should check A, B and C (airway, breathing, and circulation, respectively) before providing further care. Don't forget to call first for professional help and get permission from the victim if conscious.

Example answerは巻末（付録の前）に掲載

Chapter III.

Prevention of lifestyle disease
生活習慣病の予防

1. Definition of lifestyle disease
——生活習慣病の定義

Lifestyle diseases, such as coronary heart disease, stroke, hypertension, diabetes and cancer, use to be referred to as **geriatric diseases***1 since they seemed to mainly afflict the elderly. Although these diseases do occur in older persons, they also develop in younger people, including children. Lifestyle diseases are defined as those stemming from one's personal lifestyle and habits including diet, exercise, stress, smoking and drinking. **Surprising enough***2, even obesity is included in this category. Lifestyle diseases are also known as "**silent diseases***3." This is because an unhealthy lifestyle gradually and **imperceptibly***4 causes damage to body organs and function. Symptoms often don't appear until the disease has made major advances, and it is only at that point that most persons start thinking it necessary to change their lifestyle for the better. Since the above diseases result from the accumulation of unhealthy lifestyle habits, one can lessen the chances of experiencing such diseases by adopting a healthier lifestyle. This is why these diseases are referred to as lifestyle diseases.

Early detection and treatment can often counteract further complications. For this reason, an annual checkup is recommended.

Notes: *1 成人病, *2 驚いたことに, *3 (or silent killer) 沈黙の病気, *4 (気がつかないほど) 徐々に

Dialogue

Situation:

After Betty, an overweight woman in her 60s, has a medical checkup. Mike, a physician and close friend of her husband, Jack, encourages her to change her lifestyle explaining about dietary habits and related diseases.　肥満気味の60代の婦人，ベティが人間ドックで夫のジャックの親友である医師マイクから食習慣と合併症の説明を受け，生活習慣を変えるように勧められている

Betty: I know that lifestyle diseases used to be called **geriatric diseases**. Why was the term changed to such a **vague and broad** one?　かつては成人病と呼ばれた／曖昧模糊とした名前に

Mike: Such diseases originally seemed to be **degenerative diseases** mainly afflicting elderly persons. But, recently, we've found many young people suffering from these diseases. So, we can no longer call them geriatric diseases.　主に老人が罹る退行性の病気

Betty: Don't you think the title "Lifestyle" causes people to not take such diseases seriously?

Mike: On the contrary, these diseases are also referred to as killer diseases.

Betty: How much do our day-by-day lives determine our health?

Mike: Scientific data shows clearly that today's diseases are closely related to our daily lifestyle.

Betty: What do you mean by that?

Mike: These killer diseases are **culturally conditioned** in a way, and largely self-induced by **the way we live**.　一部は民族性にも依存するが，大体は個人の生活習慣によって引き起こされる

Betty: And "high tech" medicine is still limited in dealing with these diseases?

Mike: That's right. The challenge of medicine today, **as I see it**, is to educate and motivate people to replace their **health-erosive** lifestyle with a health-enhancing one.　私の見るところでは／健康を害するような

Betty: Then, how can I change my lifestyle?

Mike: By changing your dietary habits. Most people, however, have great difficulty in decreasing their calorie intaken **let alone** maintaining a daily schedule of moderate exercise.　日常ベースでの適度な運動は言うに及ばず

Betty: You said the "killers" are culturally conditioned. If so, **how can I be free of** them?　自分だけの努力だけでは避けられないのでは

Mike: In general, we are in a cultural group where the incidence of colon and breast cancer is high, but stomach cancer low compared for instance, to Japan. But,

Chapter III. Prevention of Lifestyle Disease

	Japanese people who migrated to Hawaii and **adopted a typical American diet** began to show the same health symptoms as typical Americans.　ハワイに移住し米国の食生活に慣れた日系米国人は逆の癌発生率を示す
Betty:	In general, would you say that we are **meat eaters**, but Japanese are primarily **vegetarians?**　肉食主義者（cf. carnivore：肉食獣）／菜食主義者（cf. herbivorous：菜食動物）
Mike:	Partially yes. However, meat isn't the only **culprit when it comes to** health problems. A study in Japan showed that people living in the northern areas tended to use more salt with their meals. And, as a result, they had a relatively higher incidence of stomach cancer or hypertension than Japanese living in other areas. More recently, many Japanese **have begun to show cancer profiles** similar to Americans.　健康に関しては肉だけが悪者ではない／だんだん米国の発癌傾向に近づいている
Betty:	Is a completely vegetarian diet sufficient?
Mike:	Certainly. Strong evidence exists to support the fact that people who eat generous amounts of fruits and vegetables have a lower incidence of cancer. But vegetarians must be careful not to leave the body **starved of** basic nutritional elements. For example, animal milk provides a lot of calcium. People who don't drink milk must be sure to find an adequate substitute for getting calcium. Moreover, if you avoid all animal products, you may have an increased chance of developing **neuropathy**, since sufficient vitamin B_{12} is mainly found in animal products.　身体が基本栄養素を渇望することになる／ビタミンB_{12}が欠乏すると神経障害のおそれがある
Betty:	Anyways, what you want to say is "**Be temperate in everything**," right?　とにかく，何事もほどほどに
Mike:	Yes! "**Too much is as bad as too little.**"　**If you ask me**, an excessive **obsession with** food and diet might **end** one **up on the road** to an eating disorder such as **anorexia** or **bulimia**.　"過ぎたるは及ばざるごとし"／言わせてもらえば，過度の食事へのこだわりは拒食症とか過食症のような摂食障害の結果を招きかねない

Quiz

A. What are "lifestyle diseases"?
B. Who are more likely to suffer from lifestyle diseases?

- C. Why are lifestyle diseases so prevalent?
- D. Do you smoke or drink alcohol, why?
- E. When do you feel stress?
- F. What do you eat for breakfast?

Answers
- A. Diseases stemming from your lifestyle choices
- B. People who make poor lifestyle choices such as eating high calorific meals and not getting exercise
- C. Most people are making poor lifestyle choices.
- D. Give your personal response.
- E. Give your personal response.
- F. Give your personal response.

Relevant expressions and additional phrases

1) Qualifier　修飾（話しにあやをつける）

① **If you ask me**, lifestyle disease is a silent killer.　　言わせてもらえば

cf. **You know what**, I lost 10 kilograms in three months. (informal style)

ねえ聞いて（単なる切りだし文句）。応えはWell, **what do you know?**　ああ，そう

② **To my surprise**, I learned that lifestyle disease is a silent killer.　　驚いたことに

③ Lifestyle disease causes fatal complications. In more blatant words, **let's say** it's a silent killer.　　いわゆる

④ I don't want to develop any complications, **let alone** cancer.　　ましてや癌など

⑤ He cannot justify his injurious lifestyle, **let alone** learn to manage his health.　　言い訳はできない。まして健康管理を身につけている（動詞）なんて言えない

2) Time order　時間的順序

① He didn't appreciate his health **until** he became ill.　　病気になるまで～気づかなかった

② It is only **when** he became ill **that** he appreciated his health.　　病気になって初めて～気づいた（強調形）

③ It was **not until** he became ill **that** he appreciated his health.　　健康とはありがたいとこと思っているのは病気になってからである（強調形）

④ He felt sorry for himself **only after** he realized **that** he **had fallen** fatally ill.　　治らないと知ってはじめて惨めになった

2. Dietary habits　　　　　　　　　　——食習慣

　These days, many young people can be seen walking along at lunch time carrying a lunch box or instant cup noodles that they bought at a convenience store. Such food is convenient, indeed, but care must be taken for maintaining well-balanced nutrition. Convenience foods often lack many of the important nutrients for the body; and those who are dependent on such foods, aware of this problem, try to fill the deficit with **health supplements**[*1]. One must be aware that such health supplements cannot replace the nutrients needed from fresh fruits, vegetables and whole grains. Also, many convenience foods are high calorie and contain a lot of salt. Sodium is a component of salt that assists the tissue cells in absorbing water. Too much sodium causes the cells to swell and the blood vessel walls to thicken, increasing the blood pressure. In addition, sodium causes blood vessels to shrink, forcing the blood pressure to rise. This can cause an interruption in the blood supply, or clotting in the blood with **thrombocytes (platelets)**[*2] that **gives rise to**[*3] a localized necrotic area. Salt may also **promote**[*4] stomach cancer. The promoter is usually not itself a **carcinogen**[*5], but fosters the multiplication of damaged cells over normal ones, creating many more **initiated cells**[*6], which can also be attacked by carcinogens and damaged further. These facts are a warning that one needs to avoid an excess intake of salt. Fruits and vegetables include a lot of potassium (kalium) that stimulates the removal of sodium from the body resulting in a decrease in blood pressure.

　One **cannot fail to**[*7] grasp the importance of maintaining a good nutritional balance. One more benefit of vegetables is that vegetable fiber works to suppress rectal absorption of cholesterol and eliminate it from the body. Vegetable fiber also helps dilute the concentration of carcinogens in the colon by binding with the carcinogens and excreting them rather than allowing them to be reabsorbed into the blood.

Notes:　*1　健康補助食品（cf. 特定保健用食品：food for specified health use，厚労省に効能書き表示を許可された食品），*2　血小板，*3　その部分に限局性の壊死を**もたらす**（主に悪い結果を**引き起こす**の意味で用いられる），*4　発癌補助物質（promoter：a carcinogenic stimulus）となる，*5　発癌物質，*6　発癌物質に暴露された細胞（発癌の第一段階のイニシエーション），*7　**必ず把握しなければならない**

Dialogue

Situation 1:
After having her blood pressure taken during a medical checkup, Betty is asking Doctor Mike about how to reduce blood pressure (BP) by dietetics.
人間ドックで血圧測定の後に，ベティが医師のマイクに，食事療法でどのように血圧を下げるかについて尋ねている。

Mike: **I have just a word** for you. Hypertension is not a disease itself, but is a **cause of** most killer diseases.　ひとこと言っておきますが／万病の元

Betty: I know I must change my dietary habits - reducing the high intake of salt - but I don't understand why you recommend me (to) eat **dark yellow and green leafy vegetables?**　黄緑野菜（e.g. spinach, carrot, pumpkin, etc.）を推奨する　cf. light-colored vegetables：淡色野菜（radish, cabbage, etc.）

Mike: They include a lot of minerals such as potassium and magnesium which **prevent blood vessels from narrowing**, thus decreasing the blood pressure.　血管が狭くなる（angiosclerosis：血管狭窄）のを予防し，血圧を下げる

Betty: Isn't it easier to take such minerals from **nutrient supplements?**
栄養補助食品

Mike: It's not always safe, or **can even be** harmful. When you take excessive calcium for healthy bones, surplus **calcium will be deposited** in the vascular walls.　害になることもある／石灰沈着（calcific deposition）となる
For this reason, you should take magnesium at the same time keeping the **intake ratio of calcium to magnesium** below two for best results. Some vegetables include both minerals and can naturally **control** the ratio and **help reduce** the chance of **ischemic heart disease**.　カルシウム／マグネシウム摂取比／このことを調整する／虚血性心疾患

Betty: It's controlled by a **provision of nature, isn't it?**　自然の摂理で制御されるわけですね

Mike: Some people **appreciate** vegetables as a gift of God.　神の恵みとありがたがる

Betty: Why do you especially **recommend** me **take** beans?

Mike: Beans include a very high quality protein, and help decrease **lipids** in the blood which leads to hypertension.　血中の脂質を下げる

Chapter III. Prevention of Lifestyle Disease 53

Betty: How do you evaluate their quality?
Mike: The quality is evaluated by a **protein score**. It is an indication of what percent of protein can actually be used by the body, excluding the unnecessary components and yet reserving **essential amino acids**. 　蛋白価／必須アミノ酸
Betty: Can we be well-nourished without eating meat?
Mike: **By and large**. Soy, also known as the **meat of the field**, is an excellent protein source. 　大概は／大豆は畑の肉と呼ばれる
Betty: I heard that fish oil doesn't raise blood pressure and, even, causes it to drop in certain cases.
Mike: Certainly. Fish includes the quality protein **taurine, or sulfur**. It helps suppress the activity of the **sympathetic nervous system** which plays a role in raising blood pressure. In the process of metabolism, fish protein is **broken down into** sodium and secreted into the urine. 　タウリンは血圧を上げる交感神経（c.f. parasympathetic nervous system：副交感神経系）の活性を抑制する／〜に分解される

Eating is a pleasure we all enjoy, yet we must be careful to avoid strong **likes and dislikes**. 　極端な好き嫌い
Betty: Does the **taurine so-and-so**, you just mentioned, only exist in fish?
　タウリンとか何とかやら
Mike: Some vegetables also include it. Physical exercise **is said** to produce taurine in the body but the **mechanism of production** remains unknown.
　と言われてる（他人の意見）／発生メカニズム（機序）
Betty: Are there any medicines for suppressing blood pressure?
Mike: Yes there are. **Suppressors** known as α β **adrenergic blocking agents** are used as medicine for expanding arterial walls **according to severity (fig. 1)**.
　α β遮断薬として知られている神経抑制剤（sympatholytic agents：交感神経抑制剤）が血管を拡張する薬（vasodilator：血管拡張剤）として症状（**重篤度**）に応じて使われる

If the nerves are stimulated, they promote the flow of calcium into the heart cells causing higher blood pressure. Then, a **calcium antagonist** is often used as an **immediate-effect agent** (magic bullet) for decreasing the BP.
　カルシウム拮抗剤／即効剤として
Betty: Is it true that good dietary habits reduce the chance of cancer onset?

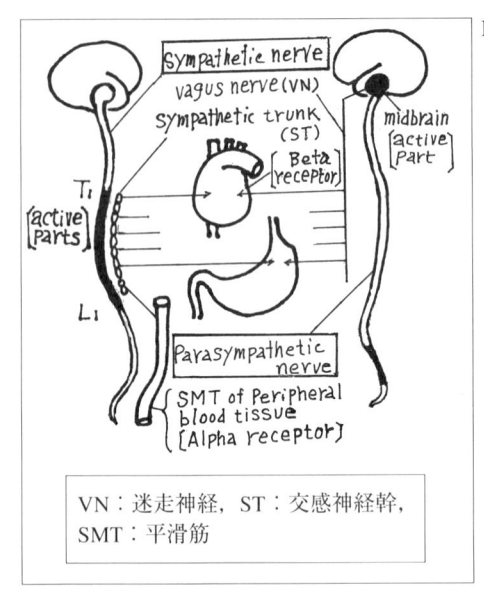

Fig.1 Automatic nervous system
自律神経系

The sympathetic nervous system has alpha and beta receptors. Stimulation of the alpha receptor causes constriction of the smooth muscle tissue (**SMT**) of peripheral blood vessels, resulting in hypertension. Alpha-blockers work against alpha receptors for relieving stress-driven hypertension. Beta receptor stimulation causes the heart muscle to constrict and increase **cardiac output**. Beta-blocker is the primary agent for relieving hypertension associated with **ischemic cardiac diseases**.
心拍出量／虚血性心疾患,

VN：迷走神経, ST：交感神経幹, SMT：平滑筋

Mike: The registered dietician, Carol, can tell you about that **in depth**. I heard that her doctoral dissertation was entitled, "Reducing Cancer Onset by Changing Dietary Habit."　詳しく教える

Quiz

A. What is wrong with convenience foods?
B. Why is too much salt harmful?
C. How does vegetable fiber help the body?
D. What is a benefit of dark yellow and green leafy vegetables?
E. Why are beans recommended?
F. How does eating fish contribute to good health?

Answers

A. Convenience foods, often lack important nutrients, are high in calories and contain too much salt.
B. Sodium, a component of salt, assists the tissue cells in absorbing water into the cells. Too much sodium causes the cells to swell and the blood vessel walls to thicken, increasing the blood pressure. In addition, sodium causes blood vessels

to shrink, forcing the blood pressure to rise. This can cause an interruption in the blood supply, or clotting in the blood.
C. Vegetable fiber works to suppress rectal absorption of cholesterol and eliminate it from the body; in addition, it helps dilute the concentration of carcinogens in the colon.
D. They include a lot of minerals such as potassium and magnesium which prevent blood vessels from narrowing, thus decreasing the blood pressure.
E. Beans include a very high quality protein, and help decrease lipids in the blood which leads to hypertension.
F. Fish includes the quality protein taurine, or sulfur, which helps suppress the activity of the sympathetic nervous system, thus playing a role in suppressing blood pressure.

Situation 2:

After making an appointment with Carol, the registered dietician, Betty goes and asks her about the kind of dietary habit that would inhibit the onset of cancer.
アポイントメントをとった後，ベティは管理栄養士のキャロルのオフィスを訪ね，どのような食習慣が発癌の発生を少なくするかを尋ねる。

Betty: Is it true that vegetables help protect us from cancer ?
Carol: Yes, to a certain level. Vegetables include a variety of vitamins. Vitamin C and E, coupled with an enzyme, defend the body from **free radicals**. These vitamins work as **free-radical scavengers** taking the place of **antioxidants**.
ビタミンCやEは酵素との共同作用で**遊離基**から身を守る／**抗酸化薬**の代わりとなって遊離基の**掃除屋さん**として働く
Betty: Oh, you're using medical **jargon** that is way **out of my realm** of understanding.　　**専門用語**（medical jargons）の羅列で，まるで**別世界の言葉**を聞いているよう
Carol: Then, let's focus on **active oxygen** as the most suspicious **initiator of carcinoma**.　　活性酸素／癌誘発因子
If oxygen in the tissue **is exposed to** excessive stimuli, it is **excited** or **activated** into active oxygen.　　過度な刺激に**暴露される**と，**励起**，あるいは**活性化されて**

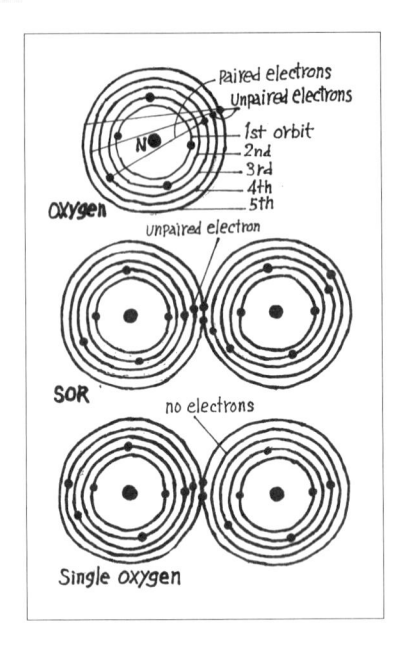

Fig.2 Oxidation reaction caused by active oxygen
活性酸素による酸化反応

If an oxygen molecule (combined with a pair of the atoms in the tissue) is exposed to excessive stimuli (Top), it is excited or activated into mild toxic **active oxygen** (SOR) (Middle). SOR can exist only in the **passing state*** in molecular form since it has an unpaired electron in one of the electron orbits. It soon attacks or deprives a surrounding normal cell of an electron. This **free radical or oxidation reaction** can end up with a very toxic **single oxygen**, a potent carcinogen (Bottom).

*準安定状態（metastable state）

注：図の詳細説明は章末の Exercise 2 を参照

It's so active that it soon attacks the surrounding normal cells leaving there a notorious byproduct known as "fatty rust" or **lipid peroxide**.　脂肪の"さび"または**過酸化脂質**として悪名高い副産物

Lipid peroxide, also known as a **free radical**, is very belligerent and also attacks **cell membranes**. It can further attack the genetic material (DNA) inside a normal cell and cause a **mutation** to occur, that could trigger the **development** of a carcinoma.　遊離基は非常に好戦的で，**細胞膜**を攻撃し，さらに遺伝子物質を攻撃して**突然変異**を起こし，癌を**誘発**する要因ともなる

Arterial sclerosis can also be caused by free radicals. **Surprisingly enough**, free radicals are even capable of impairing certain cells in the **central nervous system** (CNS) that could lead to mental disorders such as Alzheimer's disease.　動脈硬化／驚いたことに，**中枢神経**の特定の細胞にも損傷を与えアルツハイマー型のボケの原因にもなる

To be precise, the cell membrane contains **saturated** and **unsaturated fatty acid** in **phospholipids**, as its main component, to maintain a certain level of rigidity. When the unsaturated fatty acid is exposed to active oxygen, the free

	radical reaction turns it into **lipid peroxide**, even though the amount is said to be very small.　　正確に言えば，細胞膜はある程度の堅さを保つために，その主成分である**リン脂質**のなかに**飽和脂肪酸と不飽和脂肪酸**を含んでいる／不飽和脂肪酸が活性酸素に暴露されると，このフリーラジカル反応により，リン脂質はわずかではあるが**過酸化脂質**となる
Betty:	Wait a minute, please. What is "free radical **so- and- so?**"　　"遊離基とか，なんとかやら"
Carol:	The free radical reaction **might better be called an oxidation reaction** (**Fig.3**).　　酸化反応と言ったほうがよいかもしれない
Betty:	What, then, are the stimuli?　Give me a more specific example, please.
Carol:	There are many, such as heat, ultraviolet rays, x-rays, chemicals in water and food, compounds in cigarette smoke and other polluted air. Let me take ultraviolet rays as an example, since you can see the **aftermath of a free radical reaction** with your own eyes. But **remember that** it's only "**one of such reactions.**" Actually, in this case, we can not **isolate a single culprit**. フリーラジカル反応の**被害**／ただしこれは**ひとつの要因にしか過ぎないこと**を断っておく／**単独犯を特定することはできない**
Betty:	Usually, many causes are combined in the development of a carcinoma.
Carol:	Yes. Suppose you were excessively exposed to ultraviolet rays and nothing happens except that your face is tanned, or maybe even sunburned. The tanning (or burning) is caused by UVB or short-wavelength UV and may **give rise to squamous cell carcinoma** after a long **latent period**. It is a well-known **cause and effect** example because the past three American presidents have suffered from such carcinoma.　　長い**潜伏期間**の後に**扁平上皮癌を引き起こす**／**因果関係**
	Some cells in the **basal layers** are damaged by repeated stimulation from UVA that can penetrate the deeper layers. And one may be sorry to some day find **melasma** or dark spots here and there on the face as one ages.
	They are the **aftermath** or evidence of melanin that died in battle against active oxygen. But it has not yet reached the **worst scenario**. You might have **melanoma** in addition to your face losing tension and spring. 透過性の強いUVAは**基底層**の細胞を攻撃する／年をとるにしたがい，顔のあちらこちら**老人斑**（senile melanoderma：汎発性黒皮症）ができて嘆く／これはメラニンが活性酸素と戦って死んだ**結末または証拠である**／まだ**最悪**

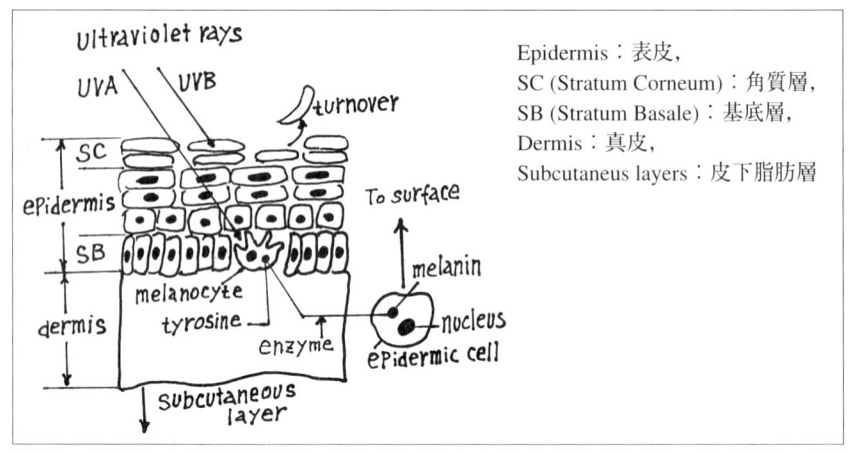

```
ultraviolet rays
UVA   UVB                turnover
     SC
epidermis                To surface
     SB                     melanin
        melanocyte
        tyrosine              nucleus
dermis   enzyme        epidermic cell
        subcutaneous
            layer
```

Epidermis：表皮,
SC (Stratum Corneum)：角質層,
SB (Stratum Basale)：基底層,
Dermis：真皮,
Subcutaneus layers：皮下脂肪層

Fig.3 Mechanism of melanin production due to ultraviolet ray exposure and layers of skin affected by overexposure.
紫外線によるメラニン生産機構と過曝露による皮膚層の被害

Ultraviolet radiation activates **tyrosine** in **melanocytes** to change into melanin, with the assistance of an enzyme, and enter the **epidermic cells**. Active oxygen is said to promote this process. Over about a month's time, these cells move up to the surface of the skin, resulting in dark spots. Note that the burns are classified by depth in emergency from first to third degree according to how far the damage extends in the main three layers. The deeper the burn, the higher the grade.
　　チロシン（メラニンの前駆体）／メラノサイト（色素形成細胞）／表皮細胞

　　　　　　　　　の筋書きが残っている／肌に張りや弾力がなくなるのは別としても，**黒色腫ができるかもしれない**

Betty:　　Isn't it a **natural aging process?**　　　当然の老化現象
Carol:　　Not really. Can't you recognize the difference in melasma among individuals? Why is there such variation? It shouldn't simply be called part of the natural aging process any longer. It's true that some melasma **is subject to** genetic or aging factors, to be sure; but most **originate from** the **natural outcome of one's own action or lifestyle.** Anyhow, there is no chance of us stopping the aging process, so **let's grow old gracefully**.
　　　　　確かに遺伝的または老化現象にもよる／ある程度は自業自得にも因る／どうせ老化は避けられないものなら優雅に歳をとろう（educated women のモットー）
Betty:　　Is there **no way of** avoiding the ugly black spots?　　　仕方のないことか

Carol: Recently, I've heard some cosmetic companies claim that the spots can be controlled by face cream with vitamin C inducers. Since vitamin C **by itself** cannot break through the skin barrier to reach deeper tissue, it must be combined with a certain **inducing agent**. Induced Vitamin C is said to prevent the **precursor** of melanin from growing. Vitamin C also helps maintain beautiful skin along with vitamin E.　ビタミンC**単独**では皮膚の防御壁を突破できない／誘導体／メラニンの**前駆体**の成長を妨げる

Betty: How does vitamin C protect the skin cells?

Carol: **All that I can say** now is that vitamin C **wards off** active oxygen and carcinogens by itself, or in combination with revived vitamin E which was once **oxidized** but **reduced** by receiving electrons from Vitamin C. If stimuli further attack damaged skin, skin **turnover** is disturbed and **keratinization** will occur. The damage to epithelial cells may lead to skin cancer. There is usually a prolonged period of time between the first cell damage and actual tumor development - **a matter of** years or even **decades** in most cases.　いま言えるのは，ビタミンCは単独で活性酸素や発癌物質を**追い払う**か，いったん**酸化**したビタミンEに電子を与えて**還元・復活**させて，共に活性酸素と再び戦わせるというだけ／皮膚の**新陳代謝**が妨げられたり，**角質化**が生じる／この**上皮細胞**の損傷が皮膚癌を誘発する／最初の細胞被害から癌の発生まで，大体は数年とか，あるいは**数10年**という期間がある

As long as one breathes, or body tissue is subject to **constant metabolism** (e.g. basal metabolism), active oxygen **will never fail to** be generated. It usually protects cells from viruses or microorganisms; but if an excess amount is present, it adversely attacks the cells, leading to coronal ischemic disease or cancer damaging the nucleus where DNA and RNA exist.　人間が呼吸をし，組織が**常に代謝**をするかぎり（例えば，基礎代謝），活性酸素は**必ず発生する**

Betty: How can I reduce the chance of producing excess active oxygen?

Carol: The best way is to eat a lot of colorful vegetables, containing the important scavenger, vitamin C, that cleans outside the cells and assists some important enzymes. Such vegetables also contain the essential Vitamin E that enforces the power of enzymes inside cells to protect against harmful active oxygen. In addition, **research shows** that moderate exercise also helps control levels of active oxygen, in contrast with smoking, stress and more **over-**

	ly-vigorous exercise.　　適度の運動が活性酸素の**発生を抑制する**というこ とは，**学問的に証明されている**／過激な運動
Betty:	Then, there's nothing to be afraid of **if only** I eat a lot of vegetables?　　十 分な野菜さえとれば
Carol:	It's not quite that simple. Some **herbs**[*1] contain nitrate due to contamination from **chemical fertilizer** or **nitrogeneous compounds**. The **nitrate turns into nitrite** while the vegetable is stored in a refrigerator or being cooked, generating active oxygen as a carcinogen. **In other words**, fresh vegetables are safer than cooked or **discolored ones**. You'll notice it when you see vegetables or salad oil change in color **over time**.　　葉菜類によっ ては**化学肥料**または**窒素化合物**で汚染されたものがあり，冷蔵庫に保存し たり，料理で加熱すると**硝酸塩**が**亜硝酸塩**になり発癌物質としての活性酸 素を生じる／つまり，新鮮な食物のほうが**変色した**ものより安全／野菜や サラダ油が，**時間が経つにつれ変色する**
Betty:	Are vegetables beneficial only for the skin?
Carol:	What I have just explained to you is one **cognitive** example only. What I wanted to say is that vitamin C helps **ward off** stomach cancer by defending the stomach from very potent carcinogens called **nitrosamines**. They are formed in the stomach from nitrates and nitrites, which are present in many foods, water, and even in saliva. Vitamin C can actually stop the formation of nitrosamines.　　目視できる1例であると断ったはず／ビタミンCは胃が んから**身を守る**／ビタミンCは**ナイトロサミン**と呼ばれる強力な発癌物質を 攻撃して胃を守る
Betty:	How do you connect skin cancer with stomach cancer?
Carol:	The skin cells that line the stomach are **originally** the same as the skin cells covering the body exterior[*2].　　胃の壁を覆っている細胞は，**起源**は体を覆 っていた細胞と同じである
Betty:	Is there a good way to select healthy foods among so many?
Carol:	Try to select **organic vegetables** or **vegetables in season** raised by reliable farms. Read **food labels** and see if **traceability** is verified - especially for **processed foods** - including a clearly written **place of origin, ingredients, additives** and **expiration date**. The **expiry date** on a package doesn't mean that the food is unedible **after that date**, but try to select **as fresh as possible goods**[*3].

有機野菜／旬の野菜／食品表示／追跡可能性／加工食品／**産地**や**成分，添加物**や**賞味期限**が明記されている／期限切れ

Notes: ＊1 cf. edible herbs：（例：白菜），edible (esculent) roots：根菜類（例：大根），nuts：堅果類（例：くるみ）

＊3 During **embryonic development**, the skin cells, dermis, stemming from the mesoderm extends inside the mouth lines the stomach and continues through the digestive tract, ending up at the anus. Cells lining the digestive cavities change their roles over the course of **development**, but **remain as epithelial cells**.

胚子期に，被蓋上皮（真皮）は**中胚葉**に由来し，口から胃部へと消化管を通して伸びて肛門で終わる。腔内の被蓋細胞は**発生**の段階で役割を変えるが，**上皮細胞**の名を留めている。

＊3語順に注目

Quiz

A. How do vegetables protect us from cancer?
B. What is active oxygen?
C. Describe a free radical.
D. Name some stimuli for creating free radicals.
E. What is melasma?
F. How does Vitamin C protect skin?

Answers

A. Vegetables include a variety of vitamins, such as Vitamin C and E, that, coupled with an enzyme, defend the body from free radicals. These vitamins work as free-radical scavengers taking the place of antioxidants.

B. If oxygen in the tissue is exposed to excessive stimuli, it is excited or activated into active oxygen. It becomes so active that it soon attacks the surrounding normal cells leaving there a notorious byproduct known as "fatty rust" or lipid peroxide.

C. A free radical, also called lipid peroxide, is a byproduct of active oxygen attacking surrounding cells. It also attacks the surrounding normal cells, as well as cell membranes. It can further attack the genetic material (DNA).

D. There are many, such as heat, ultraviolet rays, x-rays, chemicals in water and food, compounds in cigarette smoke and other polluted air, etc.

E. Melasma are dark spots appearing here and there on the face as one ages. They are the aftermath or evidence of melanin that died in battle against active oxygen.

F. Induced Vitamin C is said to prevent the precursor of melanin from growing. It helps maintain beautiful skin along with vitamin E by warding off active oxygen and carcinogens, as well as cleaning outside the cells and assisting some important enzymes.

Relevant expressions and additional phrases

1) Idiomatic parenthesis　　慣用的挿入句

1. There are few errors, **if any**, that are unforgivable.　　間違いはごくわずかで，あったにしても，無視できる。
2. She can hardly, **if ever**, understand it by herself.　　理解できるとしても，1人ではまず無理だ。
   e.g. I seldom, if ever, go there.　　そう思っても，行くのはまず無理だ。
3. Please select vegetables in season - **in short**, as fresh as possible.　　旬の野菜，つまり，できるだけ新鮮なものを選びなさい（or, in other words）

2) Hyphenated words　　ハイフン連結用語

1. Don't use the chemical jargon "free radical" **so-and-so**.　　フリーラジカルとか何とかという化学専門用語を使わないで
2. The course requires four and a half months of **on-the-job-training**.　　その学科では，4か月半の**現任教育**が必要である
3. The economy is so slow that there is only **a one-in-three chance for job-seeking students**.　　経済の低迷で，学生の**就職採用率**はたった3人に1人の割合だ
4. The government's **head-in-the-sand** policy on asylum-seekers has dealt a blow to Japan's reputation.　　亡命希望者に対する**弱腰外交**は日本の評判を損ねている（The Daily Yomiuri より）
5. The authorities stepped up guard patrols around Western embassies to ward off **would-be** refugees.　　当局は，**自称**亡命希望者を欧州の大使館に寄せ付けないように警備活動を強化した（Jiji-AFPより一部改変）
6. It's well established that confidence in a treatment can have **a mind-over-body effect** on how well the treatment works. (The Washington Post：Placebo Effects) 治療への信頼が，その効果に**心理学的影響**を及ぼすことは周知の事実である

3) Infinitive and root verbs　　不定詞と原形動詞

1. Some vegetables naturally **control** the ratio and **help reduce** the chance of the dis-

ease.

  @ **to** naturally **control** the ratio 分離不定詞（split infinitive）

  @ **help reduce** the chance 原形不定詞（bare infinitive）前置詞 to が不要

以下の命令や提案の場合も動詞は原形となる。

2 The law regulates that food labels **be** put in a clearly visible place. [= (should) **be**]

3 She suggests that one **take** well-balanced meals. (= **should take**)

3. Smoking   ——喫煙

 Smoking impairs the blood stream by accelerating **arterial sclerosis***1 resulting in elevated blood pressure. The damage on blood vessels can lead to coronary heart disease or **ischemic heart disease***2 such as angina pectoris or **myocardial infarction***3 that are associated with **hypertension***4. Today, it has been proven that smoking causes pulmonary disease, hepatic cancer, **osteoporosis***5, etc. Japanese tobacco control measures lag far behind the United States and other developed countries where the number of smokers has substantially decreased. The United States and other Western countries mandate that tobacco companies put warnings on cigarette packaging clearly stating the danger of smoking regarding disease and death. While in Japan mild warnings state something like the following: "Don't smoke too much, it may impair your health." Even more surprising is the fact that some medical personnel, who should be proponents of health, often smoke in their workplace. If you smoke, let's try to quit before you become **nicotine dependent***6.

Notes: *1 動脈硬化症, *2 虚血性心疾患, *3 心筋梗塞, *4 高血圧, *5 骨粗鬆症, *6 ニコチン依存症（cf. alcohol dependence：アルコール依存症）

Dialogue

Situation :

    Betty tries to get Jack to stop smoking by telling him what she has recently learned about the dangers of passive (second-hand) smoking and the well-documented fact that smoking leads to many killer diseases.

    ベティがジャックに，最近おそわった受動喫煙の恐ろしさと，喫煙がすべての致命的な病につながる事実を話して禁煙させようとしている。

Betty: I don't want you to smoke in this room. A **whiff of tobacco** makes me sick. Besides, **second-hand smoke** contains hundreds of toxic agents. You know some of them are proven carcinogens that directly affect the laryngeal region and lungs. Didn't you see today's newspaper?　タバコのにおい／副流煙

Jack: What did it say?

Betty: It says, "Statistics show that **passive smoking** from parents causes children to be **a bit slower in class**." I think it's **partially because of** your smoking that our son **didn't make it into** the school that we expected. Passive smoking also affects a **developing embryo**. Oh, that reminds me! His wife **is expecting**. The **baby is due** this summer. I pray that the baby won't be **born prematurely** because of his smoking. **Like father, like son,** indeed!
受動喫煙／成績が悪い／責任の一部がある／期待はずれ／発生段階の胎児／おめでた／出産予定日／未熟児／この親にして，この子あり

Jack: Are you blaming every problem and concern on my smoking? Uh, **if you'll excuse** my personal opinion, smoking has been **a part of class and culture** for many generations.　～を言わせてもらえば／長年にわたる**階層文化**

Betty: **Give me a break**, will you? Are you trying to **infer** that smoking symbolizes elitism and sophistication? Who is it that took five years to graduate?
冗談よしてよ／喫煙が上流階級の象徴とでも**言うつもり**

Jack: Ok. I'll give up smoking here and go **take a puff** in my room.　一服する

Betty: You're hopeless! You don't realize how it damages your health.

Jack: When did you become an expert on tobacco control?

Betty: You should have attended the community anti-tobacco campaign meeting. A panelist said that smokers suffer from many problems, and he warned the audience by asking, "Can you imagine your lungs being turned black with tar? Tar causes bronchi disorders, **chronic bronchitis** and **asthma**. How distressing it is to have the air passages blocked because of narrowed **bronchiolus** and increased mucus secretion. Lung cancer is the final destination of smokers." Another panelist stated that the chance of a smoker developing lung cancer is much higher than a non-smoker's. In addition, passive smoke increases the chance of lung cancer among family members 20 to 30 percent compared to a nonsmoker's family. The sufferer seems to have difficulty breathing **with less and less** air space in the lungs - as if he **were drowning**.
タールで**慢性気管支炎**や喘息のような気管支の異常が生じる／**細気管支**が

細くなったり粘液が増えて気道が詰まると，どれほど苦しいか／肺の空気がだんだん少なくなって／まるで**溺れている**みたいに

Jack: You are scaring me as if you were Doctor Mike.

Betty: I heard that nicotine constricts the arteries. Also, If one smokers a pack of cigarettes a day, the incidence of ischemic heart diseases is said to be **as much as** 20 times higher **than** a non-smoker. Most other cancers, besides lung cancer, are connected to smoking - cancer of the esophagus, stomach, liver, and even in the **cervix of uterine**, etc. etc. Moreover, it has an effect on ED (erectile dysfunction) as well. 喫煙者の虚血性心疾患の発生率は非喫煙者の20倍も**高い**らしい／**子宮頸部**にさえ

Jack: You're kidding!

Betty: For women, especially around my age, smoking is a cause of **osteoporosis**. 骨粗鬆症の原因のひとつ

Jack: What is the "osteo" so and so?

Betty: **I hear that it is** a marked loss of bone density and, **in turn**, increase in hollow space (**bone porosity**) in bone mesh (**bone trabeculae**). Many elderly women who get a bone fracture at the neck of the thigh bone (**femoral neck**) tend to become **bed-ridden***, followed by **senile dementia**. Don't you think it **devastates quality of life** for the rest of a woman's life? **Life quality** seems more important than **life quantity**, don't you think?
聞くところによると，骨密度がうんと減って，**続いて**骨の網目（**骨梁**）の間がスカスカになる（**骨有孔化**）／太ももの根元（**大腿骨頸部**）が折れて，**寝たきり**になって**老人性痴呆症**が起きる／余生の**生活の質**を台なしにする／大事なのは**健康寿命**で，ただ**長生き**すればよいものではない

Jack: Yes. I think so. Why is an older woman **likely to come down with** the disorder? 陥りやすい

Betty: When I visited Mike for the results of **my check-up**, he said, "It's a kind of menopausal disorder. For **menopausal women**, bone metabolism works well in maintaining bone density balance - where old bone cells are broken down by **osteoclasts** and replaced with new cells by **osteoblasts**. Once menstruation ceases, a woman becomes more **prone to** osteoporosis because levels of the female hormone (**estrogen**), that helps keep bones absorbing calcium, decreases." 婦人科検診／閉経時女性／破骨細胞／骨芽細胞／陥りやすい／エストロゲン

Jack:	Is there any way to slow the **aging process**?　その**老化現象**を遅らせる
Betty:	Mike said, "Stimulation to bones helps create a protein (**cytokine**) which serves to stimulate production of the repairing cells that, in turn, promote the absorption of calcium in the bones." He also stated that a kind of hormone responsible for calcium level in the blood is produced from vitamin D. These two factors **combined to create** a strong bone. **Surprisingly enough**, sunshine produces vitamin D. I also learned from Dr. Mike that the skin (**subcutaneous fat**) includes the **precursor** of vitamin D, and sunshine helps turn it into vitamin D. Did you know that vitamin D is known as a sunshine hormone?　サイトカイン／相俟って／驚いたことに／皮下脂肪／前駆体
Jack:	That's news to me; but I can guess what he told you next. Try to walk and expose yourself to moderate sunshine as much as possible.
Betty:	That's right. He said that walking or jogging in mild sunlight helps stimulate the absorption of calcium into the bones. While walking, bones **subtly expand and contract**, stimulating bone metabolism. That is why walking and **basking** in the sun **work together for** the intake of calcium.　わずかに伸縮する／日光浴をする／相乗作用がある
Jack:	I understand Mike's real intentions. He well knows my bad habits. He is trying to get me to stop smoking by teaching you the effects of passive smoking. And now he's preaching about walking and basking in the sun.
Betty:	He is very kind to you.
Jack:	I feel I must quit smoking. But I know smoking stimulates the sympathetic nervous system that controls the **satiety center**. Once I stop smoking I shall **never fail to** gain weight.　喫煙は交換神経を刺激して**満腹中枢**を抑制する／禁煙をすると必ず太る
Betty:	Young women **substitute** non-calorie candies for sweets when they feel frustration from dieting. Mike said exercise also helps **ease one's appetite** by stimulating the nerves. In addition, He mentioned that many people **apply** nicotine patches **while they are off cigarettes to relieve** the nicotine dependence.　口寂しくなったときはケーキの代わりにノンカロリーキャンディで**代替する**／運動は**食欲を抑える**のに役立つ／**禁煙中**にニコチン依存症から抜け出すために多くの人がニコチンパッチを**貼る**
Jack:	Your arguments are convincing. I believe you **would have made** an excellent lawyer. But I have the **sneaking suspicion** that you **conspired togeth-**

Chapter III. Prevention of Lifestyle Disease 67

er with Mike to stop my smoking? その説得力では，立派な弁護士になれたのに／もしかして，マイクとぐるになって禁煙させようというのでは

Betty: You really are a **cynical person**. **Is that the way** you treat the kindness of others? ひねくれ者／ひとの好意をそんなふうにとらないで

Note: ＊ a bed-ridden patient 寝たきり患者 (cf. a money-oriented person：金権亡者)

Quiz

A. How can smoking lead to heart disease?
B. How advanced are Japanese tobacco control measures compared to other developed countries?
C. What are some dangers of passive smoking?
D. How does smoking affect the lungs?
E. How are smoking and heart diseases related?
F. Why is an older woman more likely to come down with osteoporosis?

Answers

A. By damaging the blood vessels
B. Japanese tobacco control measures lag far behind the United States and other developed countries.
C. Statistics show that passive smoking from parents causes children to be a bit slower in class. Passive smoking also adversely affects a developing embryo. Smoking has also been linked to a **host** of other children's health problems. 大部分
D. Smoking turns the lungs black with tar. Tar causes bronchi disorders, chronic bronchitis and asthma. The air passages gradually become blocked because of narrowed bronchiolus and increased mucus secretion. Lung cancer is the final destination of smokers.
E. Nicotine, from smoking, may increase a smoker's incidence of ischemic heart diseases is said to be level as much as 20 times higher than a non-smoker.
F. Once menstruation ceases, a woman becomes more prone to osteoporosis because levels of the female hormone (estrogen), that helps keep bones absorbing calcium, decreases.

Relevant expressions and additional phrases

1) Synergism and antagonism 相乗効果・拮抗作用

1 There is a **synergism** of cytokine and vitamin D for maintaining healthy bones.

サイトカインとビタミンDは骨を健康に保つ相乗作用がある。
② Cytokine and vitamin D **go hand in hand** to keep healthy bones.
                         work together for keeping~

③ Sympathetic and parasympathetic impulses from the automatic nervous system **are combined to regulate** the body's automatic (involuntary) functions for restoring and maintaining homeostasis. 自律神経からの交感・副交感神経インパルスは体の自動的（不随意）機能を制御し，速やかにホメオスタシスを維持・回復させる。

④ Both impulses function **in opposite** or **antagonistic** ways for adjusting and maintaining equilibrium. 拮抗して

⑤ The processes of **anabolism**, that builds food molecules into more complex chemical compounds, and **catabolism**, that breaks down complex compounds into simpler forms, **work in opposite directions**; but by doing so are able to counterbalance each other, and **together make up** (constitute) the process of metabolism. 食物分子を複雑な化学合成物質に変える同化作用（物質合成代謝）は，複雑な化合物を単純な形に変える異化作用と互いに逆方向の過程であるが，ともに代謝の過程を司る。

2) Degree of morbidity　　罹患の程度

・Smokers are more **prone to** coronary heart disease than non-smokers.

    ①   ~ likely to succumb to
    ②   ~ likely to suffer from
    ③   ~ likely to come down with
    ④   ~ likely to be stricken by

3) How to turn down softly　　丁寧な断り方

Would you mind **my** smoking here?

① I'm sorry, I would. I'm concerned about passive smoking.
② I hope you don't. I'm afraid of second-hand smoking.
③ I wish you wouldn't. I'm allergic to the smell.　　理由を述べる
④ Yes, but thanks for asking.

  cf. Yes, I do. ("***Yes***" for **refusal**, but **impolite** if spoken too strongly)
  cf. Not at all. ＜or＞ I don't mind. ("**No**" for **acceptance**)

4) Periphrastic expressions　婉曲表現

1) be **expecting**   i.e. be pregnant　妊娠している
2) monthly **period**   i.e. menstruation　生理
3) **overweight** patient   i.e. obese patient　肥満患者
4) **underweight** or slender patient   i.e. **thin** (**skinny**) patient　痩せた
5) below average height   i.e. **short** (**small**) patient　小柄な
6) **disabled in** eyesight (speech)   i.e. **blind** (dumb) patient　盲目（聾唖(ろうあ)）の

4. Stress and Depression　——ストレスとうつ病

　Stress can cause stomach or duodenal ulcer and other problems. It can also disturb sleep, leading to malfunction of the **autonomic nervous system**＊1 and immune reaction. Thus it is considered another lifestyle disease.

　Depression is a neurotic disorder **characterized by**＊2 fatigue, headache, **insomnia**＊3, difficulty in concentration, and **lack of capacity for enjoyment**.＊4 It is triggered by a deficiency of **neurotransmitters**＊5 such as **serotonine**＊6 which acts as a **vasoconstrictor**＊7, and **noradrenaline**＊8 that stimulates the **sympathetic nervous system**＊9. An Ohio State University study shows that people who **are unhappy on** ＊10 the job, not getting support or getting a lot of criticism, **are more prone to** ＊11 injury. Thus, it was shown that emotional well-being and physical well-being **are closely linked**＊12. If you find yourself becoming pessimistic and melancholic, or some of the above symptoms fit your mental condition, **manage to**＊13 find time to take a good rest and enjoy a hobby. Don't hesitate to visit a psychiatric doctor, because this is one of the diseases **common to civilization**＊14. The World Health Organization reports that **three percent**＊15 of the worldwide population, or more than a hundred million people, suffer from depression.

Notes: ＊1 自律神経，＊2 〜を伴う特徴がある，＊3 不眠症，＊4 楽しむゆとりがない，＊5 神経伝達物質，＊6 セロトニン（不安，抑うつを制御），＊7 血管収縮神経，＊8 ノルアドレナリン（or, norepinephrine：意欲・志向を制御），＊9 交感神経系，＊10 不満である，＊11 かかりやすい，＊12 微妙に影響し合っている（or, be subtly associated with each other），＊13 なんとか努力する，＊14 文明に伴う（or, be collateral with），＊15 cf. 7% in U.S. and 5% in Japan

Dialogue

Situation :

A man called John, by his first name, consults a psychiatric doctor. After the consultation, his wife is called into the office for getting advice on supporting him at home.

愛称でジョンと呼ばれる男性が，神経科医の診察を受ける。後から奥さんが自宅での支援法のために呼ばれる。

Doctor: What seems to be the problem?
John: Recently, I've been feeling fatigue and am **unable to sleep at night**.
不眠症に悩む（i.e. suffer from insomnia）
Doctor: Have you been under a lot of stress?
John: Actually, I'm a little unhappy with the current job situation. My work project team has recently been **getting a lot of criticism** from other departments.
ひどく叱られている
Doctor: You could be suffering from a mild case of depression. What other symptoms are you having?
John: Well, sometimes I get headaches, and have difficulty concentrating. On top of that, I can't **find any gratifying aspect** in my current work. I don't feel **I'm going anywhere** with my position. Also, I feel everyone around me is talking about me behind my back and looking down on me. Moreover, I'm having frequent flashbacks of bad memories of the past which make me **feel despondent**.　　なんのやりがいも感じない／このままではどうにも浮かばれない／生きていてもしようがない気がする
Doctor: You should find more time to rest and enjoy a hobby.
John: I will try to take more time for relaxing and doing activities I enjoy.
Doctor: If the problem persists, we can pursue further steps to help you. So, please don't hesitate to visit anytime. Depression is a common lifestyle disease suffered by many. According to an ABC News poll, one in every eight Americans has been treated with **antidepressants** at some stage in his or her life. The term "depression" still tends to **bring up** the image of a **demonic disease or stigma**. But this is an **archaic view**, and no longer reality.
生涯のある段階で抗うつ薬による治療を受けている／うつ病という病名は，

Chapter III. Prevention of Lifestyle Disease　71

　　　　まだ，悪魔のような病気とか汚名だとかを連想させる／古びた考え

After John came out of the office, his wife was called in.　　ジョンの後に，奥さんが呼ばれる

Doctor:　He seems to be suffering from mild depression. Today, I listened to his **complaints** and subscribed an antidepressant. Let's wait and see how it works **for the time being.**　　ご主人の様子（愁訴）を聞いて／しばらく様子をみる

Wife:　Why does he seem so **crestfallen**?　　しょげている

Doctor:　He seems to be what we categorize as a Type A person. This type of person is more **likely to come down with** this depression disorder.　　タイプAの人はこの病気に落ち入りやすい

Wife:　His blood type is certainly "O."

Doctor:　It's not blood type that I'm referring to, but type according to a standard psychological categorization.

Wife:　Are there any specific characteristics for a person in his category?

Doctor:　Yes. They tend to be very methodical, serious and almost fanatical by nature; and are **more prone to** stress than others. Does this **sound like** him?　　ストレスに対して弱い／～に心当たりがある

Wife:　Yes, indeed. He has recently been grumbling at my sloppy housework. I've become **fed up with** his attitude of trying to **find fault with** me.　　あら捜しばかりばかりする態度にうんざりする

Doctor:　He hasn't seemed to **come to terms with** his mental illness. Please keep it in mind, for both you and your husband, that depression is not simply **a matter of mood**, but a disease. It takes time to overcome it, but we can do much more than before to help thanks to advances in psychiatry.　　精神的な病気であるということを（あきらめて）受け入れようとしない／単なる気の持ちようではなく病気である

Wife:　How do you evaluate the degree of seriousness of his disease?

Doctor:　Mainly, we do a **clinical interview** based on a **MADRS rating** that was developed by a British psychiatrist. During the interview, we closely monitor the client's facial expressions and posture. There are 10 subject areas with each area rated on a 0~6 scale. For example, he would score a 6 for his apparent despondency in the area of "Appears sad and unhappy most of the time." And he might score a 2 in the area of concentration entitled, "Occasional difficulties in **collecting one's thoughts**." The higher the scale, the higher the severity. According to the MADRS rating, your husband is classified as suffering from a mild case of depression. 　問診は主に，英国の心理学者の Montgomery Asberg Depression Rating Scale, に基づいて行われる／ときたま**集中力**に欠ける

Wife: How should I deal with him at home?

Doctor: First, Never say "Do your best!" to him even in an effort to encourage him. Second, try to keep him from having to deal with making abrupt "yes" or "no" answers. It may have an adverse effect on him. Third, try not to say the words "must" or "should" to him. He may **become obsessed with** the idea of "never" or "ever", causing him additional anxiety. Such expressions sometimes **drive** this type of person **into a corner**, so to speak, by **aggravating** their mental condition. Finally, when interacting with him, stay **aloof** or **detached**, to prevent his feeling pressure and help him remain calm.
完璧さを求めて"決して"とか"絶対に"とかいう**脅迫観念にとりつかれる**／そのような言葉は病気を**悪化させ**，彼を**窮地に追い込む**／ある程度の**距離をおいて接する**

Wife: If he takes the medicine you prescribed over a long period of time, is there any possibility of him developing **drug dependence**? 　薬物依存性

Doctor: We use a so-called third generation antidepressor, **SSRI**, that is said to be much safer than previous medicine. But, for that matter, even the older medicines of this type did not cause dependence. So, you don't need to worry. On the other hand, this is a long-term disease, so you need to encourage him constantly and make sure that he takes his medicine regularly. He will improve gradually, but may still suffer cycles or **bouts of ups and downs** along the way. As long as you understand this and take care of him accordingly, everything should be alright. 　いわゆる第三世代の薬，**選択的セロトニン再取り込み阻害薬**（Selective Serotonin Re-uptake Inhibitor）を用いている／一進一退を繰り返しながら

Wife: Thank you for explaining all that to me. I think **I've got it**. When should he visit you next? 　わかりました

Doctor: In a couple of weeks from today should be fine. 　2週間後の今日です。
(i.e. on Wednesday just two weeks later, or the Wednesday after next)

Quiz
   A. What problems can stress lead to?
   B. List some symptoms of stress.
   C. How many people worldwide suffer from depression?
   D. What is good advice for relieving stress?
   E. What is a Type A person?
   F. Describe the MADRS rating.

Answers
   A. Stress can cause stomach or duodenal ulcer, as well as sleep disturbance, leading to malfunction of the autonomic nervous system and immune reaction.
   B. Fatigue, headache, insomnia, difficulty in concentration, and lack of capacity for enjoyment
   C. Three percent of the worldwide population, or more than a hundred million people
   D. Take more time for relaxing and doing activities you enjoy.
   E. Someone more likely to suffer a depression disorder according to a standard psychological categorization.
   F. A rating system, developed by a British psychiatrist, for evaluating the degree of seriousness of a person's mental illness or depression by closely monitoring the person's facial expressions and posture.

Relevant expressions and additional phrases

1) Calendar　暦
　　① a day of the week　曜日
　　② a day of the month　何日
　　③ order of dating　日付の語順　time / month / day / year / place
　　事実の記述：An atomic bomb was dropped at 8:15 am, (on) August 6, (in) 1945, (on) Hiroshima.
　　The year 1945 saw the atomic bombing of Hiroshima at 8:15 on August 6.　　1年前の今日このとき　　＠年代／時間の強調（無生物主語：文語体）
　　At 10:29 a.m. Eastern time, September 11, 2001, the first suicide hijackers launched an unprovoked attack on the World Trade Center north tower.　　TVニュースの時間報告（現在）
　　8:46 a.m....the first plane crashes into the WTC north tower...10:29 a.m....the tower

collapses.　経過報告（現在）

2) Phrasal verbs　　動詞句
- ① bring up = remind (a person) of　　連想させる
- ② come down with = contract (the flu)　　（重病に）罹る
   - cf. catch (a cold)　　（軽い病に）罹る
- ③ come up with a good idea = think of　　思いつく
- ④ put up with = bear　　我慢する
- ⑤ come to terms with = yield to　　諦めて受け入れる
   - @ Yield to pedestrians.　　（歩行者優先：交通標識）
- ⑥ find fault with = fault (a person)　　あらを探す
- ⑦ be fed up with = have enough of　　飽き飽きする
- ⑧ be obsessed with = be compelled　　脅迫される
- ⑨ get involved in = meddle in　　干渉する

3) Expression of feelings　　感情表現
a) Despondence　　落胆
- ① I feel blue.　　憂鬱だ
- ② I feel gloomy (depressed).　　落ち込んでいる
- ③ What a pity (It's too bad).　　残念だ（情けない）
- ④ **I am sorry** to have missed you.　　会えなくて**残念**だった
- ⑤ **I was disappointed** with my test result.　　試験結果をみてがっかりした
- ⑥ He was **less than** excited.　　がっかりした（disappointed）の婉曲表現（euphemism）
- ⑦ He is always **brooding**.　　いつもくよくよしている

b) Similar but different meanings　　似て非なる表現
- ① I am embarrassed.　　恥ずかしい
   - cf. He is ashamed of himself.　恥じている。
   - cf. That's a shame.　残念だ
- ② He was pleased.　　うれしい
   - cf. **I'm glad** to meet you.　　はじめまして
- ③ How I **envy** you.　　うらやましい
   - cf. I feel **more than** envy.　　恨めしい（hatefulの婉曲表現）

c) **Selecting an adjective according to the situation**　状況に応じた形容詞の使い分け

例：**old**　なつかしい

① Lately, I've been missing my **old** hometown.　最近，故郷が**なつかしい**。

② Long time, no see. All the **old familiar** faces!　お久しぶり，**なつかしい**顔ばっかり

③ Indeed, we remember the **good old** days.　ほんとうに，あの頃が**なつかしい**

　i.e. Those were the days.

④ I finally returned home for the first time in twenty years. What **nostalgic** scenery!　念願かなって20年ぶりに戻ってきた。　なんと**なつかしい**光景だろう

4) **Faultfinding**　揚げ足をとる

① He always **finds fault with** me.　あら捜しをする

② 　　　～ **trips** me **on** my own words.　揚げ足をとる

③ 　　　～ **carps at** my faults.　とがめる

④ 　　　～ **carps about** what I did.　けちをつける

⑤ 　　　～ **picks on** me.　あら捜しをする

Exercise III.

III-1. English Composition Drill

Answer in English in more than 50 words using the following given words.

Title: Why do you think it is recommended that medical staff don't smoke in front of patients?　なぜ医療スタッフは患者さんの前でタバコを吸ってはいけないのか

Given words: second-hand smoke：副流煙，convince a patient：患者を納得させる，demonstrate accountability to the public：社会に対して責任を全うする

III-2. English / Japanese translation

Translate the following English into Japanese referring to Fig. 2 and the technical terms below.

Active oxygen represented by **superoxide reductase** (**SOR**) is referred to as oxygen that has unpaired electrons, in an electron orbit, that are seeking to be paired with electrons from other atoms. This phenomenon of gaining electrons is otherwise called an **oxidation reaction**; and the loss of electrons, or vice versa, a **reduction reaction**. **Enzyme superoxide dismutase** (**SOD**) plays the role of turning most SOR into **hydrogen peroxide**; in turn, other enzymes also try to detoxify the SOR, but some inevitably remain. The remaining SOR get coupled with copper or iron ions in a cell where a reaction occurs to change them into **hydroradicals**, which finally react with the initiator, SOR, and turns into **single oxygen**, the most toxic oxygen. In a nutshell, the free radical reaction **might better be called an oxidation reaction**. It simply means the unpaired electron tries to deprive other shells of electrons to fill its electron orbit (See SOR in **Fig. 2**), so the reaction is more active when the orbit has no electrons (See Single Oxygen in **Fig. 2**).

Technical terms: superoxide reductase（SOR）：スーパーオキシドラジカル, unpaired electrons：不対電子, oxidation reaction：酸化反応, reduction reaction：還元反応, SOD（superoxide dismutase）hydrogen peroxide：過酸化水素, hydroradical：ヒドロラジカル, single oxygen：一重項酸素, shell：（電子軌道を持つ）殻

Example answerは巻末（付録の前）に掲載

Chapter IV.

Suggestions based on laboratory test results
検査値に基づくアドバイス

1. Hyperlipidemia due to obesity
——肥満による高脂血症

According to CBS News in America, **obesity**[*1] has surpassed smoking in becoming the number one cause of death. CBS also reported the results of a four-year study of 40,000 nurses, referring to the Journal of the American Medical Association (JAMA), that suggested even a small change in weight could have a major impact on quality of health. For example, overweight women, forty-five years and over, could handle everyday life activities better and have significantly fewer aches and pains by losing just five pounds (2 kg). Obesity results from an excess intake of energy that cannot be consumed by the body and, as a result, accumulates in **adipose tissue**[*2] or internal organs as fat. **Dysbolism**[*3] may cause an increase in fat as well. Obesity is classified into two types: **subcutaneous fat**[*4] and **intra-abdominal fat**[*5]. The latter type is more serious since it can damage **intra-peritoneal (IP)**[*6] abdominal organs. **Hyperlipidemia**[*7] is the most common problem stemming from obesity and can develop dangerous complications. It is a metabolic condition in which either level of **total cholesterol**[*8] or **neutral fat**[*9] is raised. When complications are not present, it is simply called **cholesteremia**[*10]. However, when an increased level of plasma cholesterol is found, the metabolic condition is called **hypercholesterolemia**[*11], which is associated with a high incidence of coronary heart disease and **arterial sclerosis**[*12].

Notes: ＊1 肥満症，＊2 脂肪組織，＊3 代謝異常，＊4 皮下脂肪（型），＊5 内臓脂肪（型），＊6 腹腔内の ＊7 高脂血症，＊8 総コレステロール，＊9 中性脂肪（or, triglycerides: トリグリセリド），＊10 コレステリン血（症），＊11 高コレステロール血症，＊12 動脈硬化

Dialogue

Situation:

When consulting Doctor Mike, Betty **feels too embarrassed** to ask him to repeat his explanation that she failed to understand. So, instead, she asks Carol, the registered dietician, some questions about **hyperlipidemia** and the kind of dietary habit that reduces the chance of causative diseases. 　ベティは，診察時にマイク医師の説明がわからなかったが，**気おくれして反復説明を求めることができず**，代わりに管理栄養士のCarolに**高脂血症**とその余病について説明を求める。

Betty: How does one measure obesity and determine to what extent, from a medical point of view, a remedy is needed?

Carol: The most common index is **BMI** (body mass index). When the value exceeds 25, it defines one as obese. BMI parallels the **obesity degree**. When the obesity degree is determined to be 20% or more above the standard value, it indicates obesity. 　肥満の指数**BMI**（body mass index）は**肥満度**に比例する
It is said that "A cold may develop into all kinds of illness," and **so may** obesity. 　風邪は万病のもと"といわれるが，肥満もしかりである

Betty: Why do you think I can't lose weight?

Carol: Generally speaking, overeating is the most common cause.

Betty: I don't think I eat so much at **a meal**.

Carol: Then maybe you **eat between meals**? I can hardly believe that you would be the type of person we call a "**couch potato**" as your husband Jack might happen to be. Snacks such as French fries or potato chips have a surprisingly high number of calories. Eating **late-night snacks** is the worst habit. Late at night, the parasympathetic nervous system becomes active in promoting the absorption of nutrients. It raises the blood glucose level leading to obesity. 　一度の食事（＝ドカ食いをしない）／間食／ご主人のジャックが仮にそうだとしても，あなたが**カウチポテト族**（ソファーでごろ寝しながらポテトチップスやカロリーばかり高くて栄養価の低い駄菓子=Junk foodを食べながらTVばかり見ている人）だとは思えない（armchair athleteという表現もある）／夜食

Betty: I never have any snacks between meals, **let alone** after supper. 　まして夜

食など

Carol: Then, are you on an extreme diet of **going without certain meals**? It'll promote a keener appetite at the following meal and cause **more overeating** than expected. Moreover, your fat cells develop the tendency to store more **body fat** as reserve for the next occurrence of lack of food (**skipping a meal**), as in the case of a camel's hump. In addition, skipping meals can cause ulcers in the stomach or duodenum due to excess secretion of gastric juice. 欠食する／次の食事で自然と**まとめ食い**となる／脂肪細胞はらくだの瘤のように，次の**欠食**に備えて常に**体脂肪**を蓄えようとする

Betty: **I am ashamed to admit that** I usually take brunch to skip breakfast and lunch. それを聞くと**耳が痛い**

Carol: You know the fact, don't you, that more than 30 percent of American women diet; but 90 percent of dieters will eventually regain all their weight. I recommend you start a regular exercise routine and change your dietary habits. Also, one health fact often overlooked is **quick chewing**. The **satiety center** is said to work 20 minutes after you start eating. So, even if you eat a large amount of food before it starts working you won't feel full. **Prolonged eating** also won't satisfy your appetite. Distractions such as watching TV or chatting during a meal tend to prolong the eating time. But some doctors warn that excessive dedication to increasingly strict dietary plans can leave the body starved for basic nutrition and lead one to develop an eating disorder similar to **anorexia** or **bulimia**. 早食い／満腹中枢／**ながら食い**も満腹感を味わえない／極端なダイエットは基礎栄養素の欠乏を招き，**拒食症**や**過食症**に似た摂食障害を招く

Betty: The doctor said the level of my total cholesterol was 230. Is it so high that I should be particularly concerned?

Carol: I'm not in the position where I can comment on it. Generally speaking, one who has a level over 220 **is classified as** hyperlipidemia. Also, be aware that it's not only a matter of the total level of cholesterol, but also the quality. 総コレステロール値が220以上の人は高脂血症の仲間に**入ります**。

Betty: What do you mean by quality of cholesterol?

Carol: Cholesterol plays an important role in the body in combination with the liver. But excessive cholesterol in the blood becomes a problem. Cholesterol cannot live in the blood by itself because lipid is not **water-soluble, doesn't get**

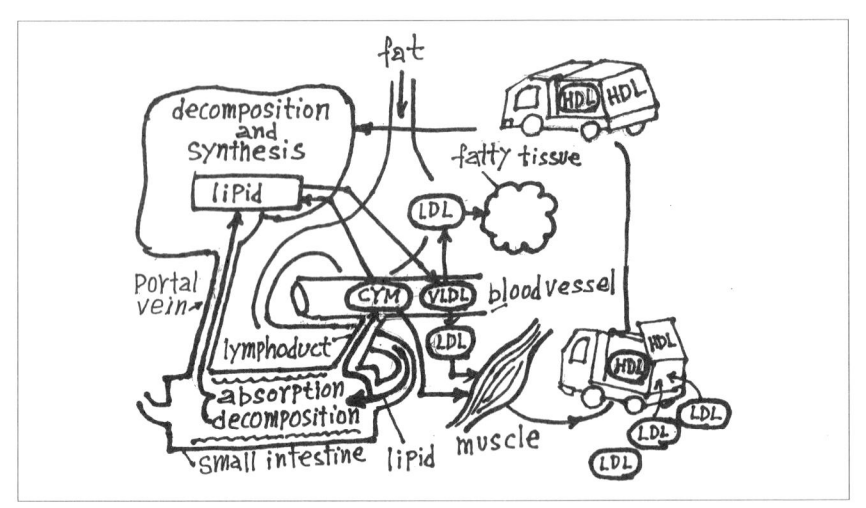

Fig. 1 Structure and metabolism of cholesterol
コレステロールの構造と代謝

Most dietary fat is ingested in the **small intestine** and carried in the blood directly as **chylomicrons (CYM)**. On the other hand, the liver turns **lipid** into cholesterol that exists as **lipoprotein** similar to chylomicrons in the blood combined with protein. On entering the cell membrane, **very low density protein (VLDL)** is **reduced** to LDL, which then enters the cell and is further metabolized releasing cholesterol. HDL combines with excess LDL and transports it to the liver, where it is metabolized and removed from circulation.
小腸／カイロミクロン／脂質／リポタンパク／超低比重リポタンパク／分解される

along with water, so it survives in the blood as **lipoprotein** by wearing a coat of protein which is **congenial to either** water **or** oil. There are two types of lipoprotein (**Fig.1**). One is called height-density lipoprotein, abbreviated as **HDL**, and the other is low-density lipoprotein or **LDL**.　コレステロールは**水溶性**ではなく水と**なじまず**／水と脂肪のどちらにもなじみやすい蛋白質の衣を着て**リポタンパク**として生き延びる／高比重リポタンパク／低比重リポタンパク

Betty: I often hear about the good type and bad type of cholesterol when I consult a doctor.

Carol: That is what I now want to mention. HDL is **protective** cholesterol **rather than being injurious**, because HDL brings excess cholesterol back to the liver where it is metabolized and removed from circulation. It works simi-

Chapter IV. Suggestions based on laboratory test results

lar to a cleaning crew (**scavenger**).
有害というよりはむしろ**有益**／HDLは余分なコレステロールを肝臓に持ち帰る**清掃員**（スカベンジャ）のようなはたらきをする

Betty: Is that why HDL is called good cholesterol?

Carol: That's right. LDL also plays an important role **as such**, bringing cholesterol to each organ. But excess LDL becomes a primary causative factor of coronary heart disease, because it dies in the arteries **leaving debris** there. It's **reluctantly called bad** cholesterol even though much of the blame lies with the person who overeats. Recent studies reveal that LDL which is degenerated or oxidized, **in plain words**, by active oxygen. So, LDL might better be called a **double-edged sword** rather than a **necessary evil**. Anyway, you need to compare LDL with HDL. If the ratio of LDL to HDL is **over three**, the chance of developing heart disease is very high (**Fig. 1**). LDHはそれなりの重要な役目を果たす／過剰なLDLは血管内で死んでそこに**残骸を残す**／**不本意ながら悪玉と呼ばれている**／本当に悪いのは活性酸素によって変性された，**ひらたく言えば**酸化されたLDLである／LDLは**必要悪**というよりは**両刃の剣**と呼ぶべき／LDL／HDL 比が3を**超えると**

Betty: My chart doesn't include the LDL value.

Carol: Usually, the LDL level is not written in the test results, but the level can be roughly estimated using the simple reduction from total cholesterol if you can remember the fact that one fifth of TG is cholesterol. Total cholesterol consists of HDL plus LDL and TG divided by five. 中性脂肪の1／5はコレステロールですので，総コレステロールはHDLとLDHの和に中性脂肪の1／5を足した値になります。通常LDHの値は検査表に書かれていませんが，TGの1／5がコレステロールであることを思えば単純な引き算でその値は概算できます

Betty: The doctor mentioned that women at my age are especially exposed to such dangers. I missed his further explanation.

Carol: You should have asked him until you understood clearly. He must have warned you about arterial sclerosis or narrowing of the vascular walls. For **post-menopausal** women or women whose **monthly period** has ended, there's no longer a need for cholesterol to produce estrogen, which is made from cholesterol. Naturally, blood cholesterol becomes more concentrated and the level of total cholesterol rises. **閉経後**または**生理**の終わった婦

人ではコレステロールが女性ホルモン（エストロゲン）を造る必要がなくなるため，結果として，血中のコレステロールが渋滞し，総コレステロール値が上がります

Betty: By the way, how is neutral fat different from **body fat**?　中性脂肪と**体脂肪**

Carol: The value determined by a blood test is for neutral fat and is written as **TG** (for **triglycerides**) on a chart. Most dietary fat, 90 to 95 percent, is ingested in a form of neutral fat, which is called "**neutral**", because it has **no electric charge**.　血液検査で検出されるのが中性脂肪で，検査表にはトリグリセライドの略でTGと書かれている／"**中性**"と呼ばれるのは**電気的に中性**だから

When one takes a lot of dietary fat or alcohol, the liver cannot work fast enough to **cover all the lipids with a protein coat**, so remaining lipids are left untouched and stored in the liver. Other surplus TG will be sent throughout the blood vessels and stored in fat cells in other organs or under the skin as body fat. Remember body fat cannot be determined by a blood test, so TG does not always run **parallel to** body fat or obesity.　肝臓はリポタンパクを造る作業が間に合わず，脂肪は そのまま肝臓に溜まる／体脂肪は血液検査では現れないので，TGが必ずしも体脂肪や肥満を**反映する**ものではない

Betty: How can I check the fat ratio? Is it different from the **said** BMI?
体脂肪は**先ほど言われた**BMIとどう違う

Carol: BMI is not enough to find out fat lying in internal organs, so called **invisible obesity**. An easy way is to check the value with a functional digital weight meter. It's a kind of **ohmmeter** or **voltameter** that measures electrical resistance of the body by letting a micro-electric current flow through it. Fat has higher resistance than that of water-contained tissue. Of course, the more fat, the higher body fat ratio you would have.　BMIは**隠れ肥満**と呼ばれる内臓内の脂肪をみつけることができない／測定機能付きの体重計は一種のオームメータや電圧・電流器で，微弱な電流を体内に流して電気抵抗を測定する

Doctors generally agree that men with more than 25 **percent body fat** and women with more than 30 percent are obese. **If only** you multiply your **current weight** by body fat percentage, you can know your **body fat mass**. For those who have excess body fat mass, diet and exercise are the standard way to reduce, but it's not an easy task. To give an example, a cup of rice has approximately 200 kilocalories, which would require one to walk one hour to burn the 200 kilocalories. Compare this number with one kilogram of body fat containing 7000 kilocalories that would require one to walk thirty-five hours.　**体脂肪率**／**現体重**に体脂肪率を掛けるだけで**体脂肪量**がわかる

Betty: How can I correctly know my body fat level?

Carol: Just step on the flat panel and watch the meter. But the reading differs each time depending on conditions, especially just after taking a bath or meal. A wet body reduces the reading. It would be better to average the measurements taken at a given time each day over a period of a week. A good time is in the evening. But, anyway, it's a rough estimation. A method to determine the precise value is obtained with an image area of fatty tissue in the **transverse-section image** scanned at the navel level. The fatty area is displayed darker than the other areas **on a CRT screen** when the image is obtained by CT scanning; and brighter using MRI. There are many ways to evaluate obesity on an image. One method determines one as obese if the fatty area occupies 100cm^2 **or more** in the image section.　　臍の位置でスキャンされた**横断面画像**／ブラウン管上に，その断面で100cm^{2}以上の内臓脂肪があれば肥満とみる

Betty: How can I reduce body fat so that I can avoid obesity-related complications?

Carol: The first step is to be temperate in everything I've told you. And never forget to maintain a well-balanced nutritional diet. Everyone knows that cultivating such a habit is a good guideline to follow, but **is easier said than done**. However, healthy habits will help one avoid the awful consequences of obesity.　　言うはやすし，されど行うは難し

Look here at this chart. You see TG as neutral fat. Oh, you need to reduce TG by 120 mg/dl. TG is mainly made from glucose **against the common belief** that the TG's root is definitely fat. So, try to take sweet foods as little as possible; or your vascular walls may rupture by being stuffed with sticky matter **similar to** an old water pipe **rupturing from the buildup of corrosion**.　　中性脂肪はその元が脂質であるという**常識とは異なり**，主にブドウ糖からできている／血管がどろどろしたもので詰まり，まるで古い水道管が詰まり**破裂してしまうようなことになる**

Betty: Oh my! How many calories, then, should I take a day?

Carol: Remember the standard weight calculated from BMI which I've already explained to you. The necessary number of calories per day is calculated with BMI multiplied by a **given index**. The index **is roughly given** according to one's activity level, with the standard as 30, and lower and upper limits of 25 and 35. Let's take **office workers** mostly engaged in **sedentary work** as an example. They would most likely be assigned an index of 25. However, if they walk more than one hour going to and coming from the office, they might receive an index of 30. In your case, as an overweight person, the index should be 25. **Physical laborers** are given 35.　　活動強度指数／大雑把には**両端の中間値**，または標準値の30を選ぶ／ほとんどが**座り仕事の事務職員**を例にとる／**肉体労働者**は35が与えられる

Quiz

A. What is the most common index of obesity and how does it define obesity?
B. What is the worst eating habit for obesity? Why?
C. What can excessive dedication to a strict diet cause?
D. Why does cholesterol exist in the blood as lipoproteins?
E. Why is HDL compared to a scavenger?
F. Why does an excessive intake of dietary fat or alcohol cause fatty liver?

Answers

A. BMI (body mass index). When the numerical value exceeds 25, it defines one as obese.
B. Late-night snacking, because the parasympathetic nervous system becomes more active late at night promoting the absorption of nutrients. .
C. It can leave the body starved for basic nutrition and lead one to develop an eating disorder.
D. Lipid is not water-soluble and doesn't get along with water; so it combines with protein, which is congenial to either water or oil, as a lipoprotein to survive in the blood.
E. HDL brings excess cholesterol back to the liver where it is metabolized and removed from circulation.
F. The liver cannot work fast enough to cover lipid with a protein coat, resulting in the uncoated lipid being stored in the liver as neutral fat.

Chapter IV. Suggestions based on laboratory test results 85

Relevant expressions and additional phrases

1) Expression of numerical formula 数式の表現

①BMI = CW(kg) / H^2(m^2) , and CW = H^2(m^2) × 22 (a BMI of 22)

Body mass index (BMI) is one of the indexes used to measure obesity. It is evaluated as current weight (CW) divided by the second power of high (H^2). Since base BMI is 22 for both male and female, a given person's weight is estimated as H^2 multiplied by 22.

②Obesity degree 肥満度

Obesity degree is calculated by subtracting the standard weight (SW) from current weight (CW), and dividing by standard weight (SW) and multiplied by 100. [(CW − SW) / SW] × 100

③Rough estimate of LDL LDLの概算法

LDL approximately equals TCH minus HDL minus TG divided by five [LDL ≒ TCH − HDL − TG / 5]. e.g., if TCH (total cholesterol) was 160 and HDL was 60. Then one fifth of a TG level of 112 would be 22.4. LDL would roughly be 77.6 which is 60 and 22.4 subtracted from 160. The ratio of LDL to HDL would be 77.6 divided by 60 or 1.3. This hypothetical level is no problem concerning arterial sclerosis since it is less than 3.

総コレステロール値TCHが160，HDLが60とすると，中性脂肪が112のとき，その1/5は22.4であるので，160 − 60 − 22.4 = 77.6であり，LDH / HDL=77.6 / 60 は1.33となり，その比が3以下であるので動脈硬化のおそれはないといわれる［160-60-22.4 = 77.6, and LDH / HDL 77.6 / 60 = 1.33］

④Barium meal concentration (S) バリウム濃度S

A given concentration of barium is calculated by the following formula.

S = [m / (m / 4.5 + a)] × 100 (%)

This reads, "S equals the result of m divided by 4.5 plus a divided into m and multiplied by 100%."

Where, S equals the concentration of barium in w/v (%), m represents mass of the barium and "a" means volume of the dissolving water in milliliter. First divide the weight of the barium by its density (4.5). This turns it into volume. This volume, added to water, makes the total volume of the barium solution. The **weight to volume percentage** is obtained by dividing the weight of the barium by the volume of solution.

あるバリウム濃度は次の式で計算されます。（式省略）ここで，Sはバリウム濃度 w／v（%），mは硫酸バリウムの重量（g），aは溶解水量（ml）です。はじめに，バリウムの重量を密度4.5で割ります。すると体積が出ます。この体積に水を加え，バリウム溶液全体の体積とします。**体積重量比**は，バリウムの重量をその溶液の体積で割って得られます

5 **Fahrenheit degrees** (F) can be converted to **Celsius degrees** (C) by the use of the formula: Celsius degrees(C) = 5/9(F-32). This reads as follows: C equals F minus 32 multiplied by five-ninths. Conversely, Celsius degrees can be obtained from Fahrenhight degrees as follows: multiply C by nine, divide by five and add thirty-two [F= (C) 9/5 + 32]. Accordingly, **normal human body temperature** is 37℃, which is equal to 98.6°F.　　華氏温度／摂氏温度／標準体温

6 Milliequivalents (mEq) ミリグラム当量

Milliequivalent (mEq) is a unit of measurement that indicates how reactive a particular electrolyte is in the body fluid. The unit, mEq, is calculated by dividing **atomic weight** (**molecular weight**) by the **valence** of an electrolyte, and the result divided by 1000. The formula is: mEq = {atomic weight (molecular weight)[g] / valence }/1000.　　原子量／分子量／原子価

7 Others　その他

・以上と超える値：forty-five years **or over**（以上），**more than** forty-five years（超える値）
・以下と未満：forty-five years **or less**（以下），less than forty-five years（未満）
・時間：Hours　one hour (1 hr), one and a half hours (1.5 hrs)
・単位：Units　two kilograms (2 kg), two hundred kilocalories (200 kcal)
　例：血糖値　a normal range of 60 to 120 milligrams per 100 milliliters [60 ~ 120 mg / 10 dl] of blood

2) Eating habits　食習慣

・be temperate in eating　腹八分　i.e. eating a little less than one desires
　cf. He always eats until he has a feeling of fullness　満腹感を味わうまで
・season food sparingly with salt　薄塩で味つけする
　cf. low-salt food　減塩食，salt-preserved foods　塩漬け
・tastes (likes and dislikes) in eating habits　食嗜好（好き嫌い）

2. Type II diabetes due to lack of exercise
——運動不足によるII型糖尿病

Lack of exercise results in obesity. This is the most common cause of diabetes that traditionally occurs in old age. This type of diabetes is classified as type II, as compared to **type I** or **insulin-dependent (juvenile-onset) diabetes mellitus**[*1]. When not specified, diabetes refers, in nine out of ten cases, to **non-insulin-dependent (or adult-onset) diabetes mellitus**[*2] which is caused by environmental factors such as overeating and lack of exercise in addition to genetic factors. According to CBS News, diabetes in children has become epidemic and the most urgent health crisis in America due to dietary habits of calorific foods. Eighty thousand new cases are added every year to the eighteen million sufferers. It has recently become a serious social issue. The lifetime cost of healthcare and lost wages for one child with diabetes is estimated to be US $ 7 million! Such children will have significant problems throughout their lifetime.

An obese person is a possible candidate for diabetes. It is a complex metabolic disorder resulting from inadequate insulin secretion which inhibits glucose uptake by cells and leads to the excretion of very large volumes of water. This accompanies the excretion of glucose in the blood or urine when the **renal threshold**[*3] is exceeded. Therefore, an increase in blood or urine glucose concentration is one of the indications of this disease. The remedy starts with **dietetics**[*4] using a diabetic diet menu which includes a minimum unit of energy (in kilograms or calories), and yet well balanced nutrients - especially avoiding a surplus intake of sugar to keep the blood sugar (glucose) level as low as possible. The other is **kinesitherapy**[*5] which is used for increasing the consumption of blood sugar. However, it is also used to prevent or remedy **hyperlipidemia**[*6] by moving large volume muscles in the body continuously over a certain period of time. Kinesitherapy is based on **aerobic exercise**[*7] which is mild enough that no lactic acid accumulates in the muscle, and so-called "air-walking that lets you smile" or jogging. All of these are common examples of moderate and sustainable exercises that can be carried out in daily life.

Notes: *1 インスリン依存性（若年発症）糖尿病（IDDM），*2 非インスリン依存性（成人発症またはII型）糖尿病，*3 腎クリアランス，*4 食事療法，*5 運動療法（ergotherapy），*6 高脂血症，*7 有酸素運動

Dialogue

Situation

        Jack, the husband of Betty, is warned by his friend Doctor Mike about his unhealthy lifestyle since he has borderline type II diabetes.　ベティの夫のジャックは境界型糖尿病であるので、友人の医師マイクに不健康な生活習慣に対する警告と脅しを受けている（友好的／インフォーマルな会話）

Mike: You seem to need some exercise, Jack.

Jack: I play golf once a week.

Mike: You better not expect to lose weight only playing golf once a week.

Jack: It's rather tough work at my age and with my busy schedule to exercise regularly.

Mike: They say, "**Where there's a will there's a way.**" You really need to find a way to exercise moderately on a daily basis.　継続は力なり

Jack: What are you trying to say, Mike?

Mike: Have you ever looked at yourself in a mirror? What a bulging stomach! You are **anything but slim**. You **can't take it easy**. You are a **true candidate** for diabetes because your blood sugar level is the same as **borderline diabetes levels**.　どうみても肥満としか言いようがない（＝スリムなんてとんでもない）／肥満を甘く見てはいけない／予備軍／境界型糖尿病

Jack: What do you mean by that?

Mike: The body has mechanisms for trying to maintain blood sugar or glucose levels within a normal range. While the normal level is within 100 to 124 milligrams per 100 milliliters for a **fasting blood glucose test**, or 140 to 199 mg/dl for **glucose tolerance test**, your levels are abnormal and remain at borderline status.　空腹血糖試験／ブドウ糖負荷試験

Jack: Wait a minute. What is the tolerance test?

Mike: If the diagnosis with the fasting blood glucose test is in doubt, sugar is given to a client orally, and the venous concentration is traced every thirty minutes. The level reached two hours following oral ingestion is called a **two-hour postprandial glucose tolerance test level**.　経口ブドウ糖負荷2時間後試験

Jack: That's probably why I had many shots after I ingested sugar water.

Mike: Try not to let the sugar levels exceed the upper limits, or you will really be

	classified as a diabetic patient.
Jack:	My blood happened to show high sugar levels because I've had to attend several parties recently.
Mike:	We have checked another indicator, HbA$_{1c}$, **to make sure**. The red blood cells slowly absorb glucose and are bound to hemoglobin to create **sugar-coated** hemoglobin (glycosylated hemoglobin), so to speak. You can make no excuse about the recent parties because this indicator reflects the glucose fluctuation **over a range of** one to two months.　念のために、エイッチ・ビー・エイ・ワン・シーを調べている／赤血球はゆっくりとグルコースを吸収してヘモグロビンと結合して、いわば**糖衣を着**たヘモグロビン（糖化ヘモグロビン）をつくる／過去1～2か月**間**の血糖変動を反映する
Jack:	Oh, I remember that I also have an inherited tendency for diabetes. My mother **paved the way** genetically.　遺伝子で**地ならしをしている**
Mike :	I've described it in the **chart**. Didn't I tell you, at your first visit, that you were in a risk group? And...　そのことは**カルテ**に書いてある
Jack:	I know what you want to say next. "Be temperate in everything," right? I've heard it before from Betty.
Mike:	**Bingo!** Look at a big cup of Coke, fries and burgers. These foods would **put** anyone **at risk**. It's a **familiar** unfortunate American tradition. But it isn't only dietary habit that is to be blamed. If you are serious about overcoming this health condition, you must keep a regular exercise routine as well. Diabetic regimens and exercise **are closely related to each other**. The important thing is to never give up. The genetic factor of diabetes **accounts for** only one-third of the risk factors. The rest are due to a lazy lifestyle and wrong food choices.　図星！（or, You can say that again）／危険に晒す／おなじみの悪習慣／糖尿病療法は食事と運動療法が**両輪**となる／遺伝による影響は危険因子の1/3を**占める**だけ
Jack:	What triggers the diabetes disaster?
Mike:	The healthy pancreas releases insulin **responsible for** the breakdown of glycogen which regulates blood sugar level. If insulin secretion is insufficient, surplus glycogen turns into **fatty acid** and is stored in the liver or in the subcutaneous layer as **neutral fat**.　健康な膵臓はグリコーゲンの代謝を**司る**インスリンを放出して血糖値を一定に保つ／インスリンが不足すると過剰なブドウ糖は**脂肪酸**となり肝臓や皮下脂肪層に**中性脂肪**として溜まる

Obesity, inactivity and aging are **all to blame for** this disease in which the body basically loses its ability to produce insulin. If you gain more weight, you need more insulin to deal with the glucose. People who get diabetes aren't able to produce enough insulin. If you take your condition lightly, **you'll pay dearly**.　すべてが（糖尿病）のもと／のんきにしているとツケが回る

Jack:　No kidding. How so?　脅かさないで。それで？

Mike:　Kidney disease may surface in the first stage. Glucose that **fails to** get into the cells is excreted through the kidneys. Because of osmosis, much water is lost along with the glucose in urination, making one thirsty.　細胞に吸収されなかったブドウ糖は腎臓から排泄される／**浸透圧**の関係で，多くの水分がブドウ糖と一緒に排尿時に失われるので，のどの渇き始める

More sever symptoms follow including circulation and vision problems leading to cardiac or cerebral stroke. Did you know that seventy-five percent of patients that develop type II diabetes die of cardiovascular disease. **Take it to heart** that **arterial sclerosis** begins at the borderline diabetes stage. But you still have time to do something about your situation.　**動脈硬化**はこの境界型の時点から始まっていることを**肝**に**銘じておく**

Jack:　I think I finally understand the **gravity of** what you're saying. Tell me, if I do develop the disease, are there any good medicines to take?
言葉の**重み**

Mike:　Various drugs and insulin are widely available for treatment, but I warn you there **is no magic pill** (wonder drug) to quickly cure the disorder which comes about as a result of neglecting one's health.　長年の不摂生で損ねてきた健康をすぐに直すような特効薬などあるはずがない

Jack:　That's **not the way to answer**, Mike, even if to a close friend.　親友だからといってもその言い方はない

Mike:　Then, try to reduce your weight first. They say, "**Prevention is better than cure.**" Why don't you start doing **aerobic exercise**? You need to keep your total cholesterol under two hundred.　転ばぬ先の杖／有酸素運動（発音に注意）

Jack:　**You've got to be joking!** I can't dance **to music**, especially at my age!
まさか！　この年で**音楽**に**合わせて踊る**なんて

Mike:　You **took it the wrong way**. Aerobics is a moderate exercise in which you

	can **concurrently** talk to another person while smiling.　勘違いしている／他人とニコニコ話しながらできる程度の緩やかな運動
Jack:	Why don't you recommend that I jog? You know I'm a good runner?
Mike:	You used to be, yes. But can you jog for more than ten minutes every day? When you jog, glucose acts as a powerful fuel to drive you for the first ten minutes. Fat replaces it thereafter. So if you want to **burn off** excess fat, you have to jog for at least twenty to thirty minutes.　余分な脂肪を**燃や**すには
	When jogging, one needs to watch their blood pulse rate (BPR) that it doesn't exceed 120bpm. One can estimate their standard pulse rate by subtracting half their age from 138 (138 - age/2). Wearing a **pedometer** may be an **incentive** for reaching one's goal for walking exercise, but don't forget to drink water whenever you **perspire** so that you can avoid **dehydration**.　万歩計を着けるとウォーキングの目標達成の**よい励み**となる／**脱水症**に気をつけて，汗をかいたときは必ず水を飲むこと
Jack:	I still don't understand why aerobic exercise is better for me than muscle exercise.
Mike:	Anyway, you should be **primarily concerned with** your weight control. Afterwards, you can start muscle exercise to avoid **muscle deterioration** and a decrease in **basal metabolism** associated with aging. The muscle is **a storehouse** where glucose is temporarily stored as glycogen after a meal so that the blood glucose level is kept constant.　とにかく，体重を落とすことに**重点を置く**／老化に伴う**筋力低下**と**基礎代謝**の低下を避けるために筋力体操をする／筋肉は食後のブドウ糖を一時的にグリコーゲンとして蓄える**倉庫**のようなもので，それで血糖値が一定に保たれる
Jack:	Wait a minute. What is basal metabolism?
Mike:	It's the minimum energy level needed to maintain one's life. One needs energy even when he or she is sleeping so that the heart and other organs keep functioning. The lower the metabolism, the less energy one needs. Now where was I? Oh yes, I was talking about blood glucose. Glucose is the **end product** of sugars (carbohydrates or starches) which are digested and decomposed in the small intestine. What is not immediately **taken up from** the bloodstream by cells is converted to glycogen and stored in the liver and muscles. Insulin secreted from the pancreas **encourages** cells to absorb more

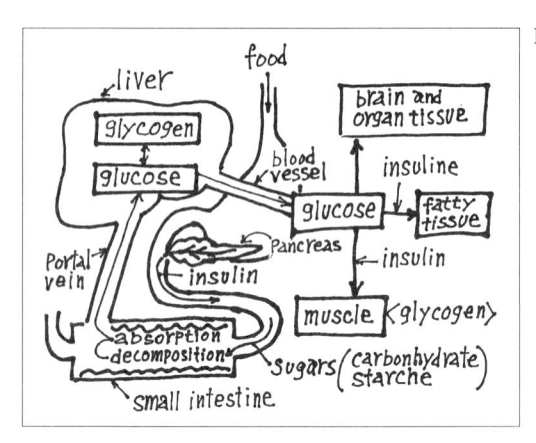

Fig. 2 Absorption and distribution of sugars
糖質の吸収と分配

glycogen **so that** the blood glucose level is lowered. When the level is low, glycogen stored in the muscles and the liver is **converted back into** glucose. Therefore, blood glucose levels elevate in cases of low insulin secretion. Also, higher blood glucose levels could mean that the lean muscle is always asking for glycogen to turn back to glucose (**Fig.2**).　ブドウ糖は糖質（炭水化物，あるいはでんぷん質）が小腸で吸収・分解されてできた**代謝最終産物**である／血流に**流入する**前に細胞に**取り込まれた**ブドウ糖は，肝臓や筋肉にグリコーゲンとして貯蔵される／膵臓から分泌されるインスリンは血糖値を下げるために細胞にグリコーゲンの吸収を**促す**／血糖値が低いときは筋肉や肝臓に保存されていたグリコーゲンがブドウ糖に**変換される**／だから血糖値が上がるのは，インスリンの分泌が悪くなっただけでなく，痩せ細った筋肉が常にグリコーゲンにグルコースに戻るように催促しているからでもある

Recent studies show that muscle promotes insulin secretion in addition to storing surplus glucose. And **muscle contraction** directly assists in glucose absorption without the help of insulin. So, you need to keep sufficient **muscle volume** to maintain a normal blood glucose level. Surplus glucose impairs the vascular walls by allowing cholesterol to **pile up leading to** sclerosis.　最近の研究で，筋肉収縮は過剰なブドウ糖を蓄えるだけでなく，それ自身がインスリンの分泌を促すことがわかっている／しかも筋肉の収縮でインスリンの助けなしに直接ブドウ糖を吸収する／だから血糖値を正常に保つためには十分な**筋肉量**が必要となる／余ったブドウ糖は血管の壁を傷

Chapter IV. Suggestions based on laboratory test results　93

つけ，そこにコレステロールが**堆積**して血管狭窄を起こす

Jack: I'm a macho, aren't I? (Jack bends his arm **with** fist **clenched** to show off his biceps).　　腕を曲げてこぶしを**握りしめ** 2 頭筋の膨らみをみせびらかす

Mike: Burn off the fat in the stomach, first, by exercising. Ask David about how to reduce the health-threatening lump of fat. He is an experienced physical therapist working at the rehabilitation department.

Relevant expressions and additional phrases

1) **Huge numbers**　　大きな数字

Ten thousand: 1万，　Hundred thousand: 10万，　Million: 100万，　Ten million: 1000万，
Hundred million: 1億，　Billion: 10億，　Trillion: 1兆，
Quadrillion（one thousand trillion）: 千兆

1. One in three, or **58 million**, American adults are overweight (defined as having a body mass index of 27.3 or more for women and 27.8 or more for men). （20〜74歳）の大人の3人に1人，または**5800万**の米国人が肥満である。

2. Obesity accounts for **$22.2 billion**, or 19 percent, of the total annual costs of treating heart disease.　　肥満は，心臓病に要する年間総費用のうち**222億**ドル，または19％を占める。

3. Japan has a population of **a hundred and twenty million**.　　日本の人口は**1億2000万人**である。

4. Japan's population is expected to fall to about **100 million** in 2050 after hitting a high of **127.74 million** in 2006; and will fall to half that amount, or 64.14 million, by 2100, according to an estimate by the Health, Labor and Welfare Ministry.　　日本の人口は2006年に**1億2774万人**のピークに達した後，2050年にはおよそ**1億人**まで減少し，2100年には半分の**6414万人**まで落ちるだろうと厚生労働省は予測した。

5. According to the United Nations, the world population that was **2,519,500,000** in 1950 increased to **6,056,720,000** by 2000, and is estimated to soar to nearly **10 billion** by 2050.　　1950年に**25億1950万**（two billion, five hundred nineteen million, five hundred thousand）人だった世界の人口は，半世紀の間に**60億5672万人**となり，2050年までにはおよそ**100億人**（ten **billion**）まで上昇すると国連は予想している。

6. Health insurance organizations refused to pay about ¥ **100 billion** to medical facilities for about **21.2 million** cases of unnecessary prescriptions and medical examinations in fiscal 2001, Health, Labor and Welfare Ministry officials said on the 27th.

厚生労働省は27日，2001会計年度に，健康保険組合が病院など医療機関に約**2120万件**の不要な投薬や検査などがあったとして，**約1000億**円の支払いを拒否したと公表した。

[7] The nation's medical expenses, which are growing due to an aging society, came to about ¥**26.4 trillion in** the fiscal year 2000.　　国民医療保険費は高齢化の進展で，2000年会計度で約26兆4000億円程度に膨らんでいる。

[8] The nation's individual financial assets totaling ¥**1.42 quadrillion**, and Japan's net assets abroad which stand at ¥**120 trillion**, are used up.　　国内の個人資産は**1420兆円**に達し，対外純資産のうち**120兆円**が消費された（The Daily Yomiuri改）。

[9] As one **quadrillion** equals **one thousand trillion**, one quadrillion yen could be exchanged into ten trillion dollars, if the yen to dollar exchange rate was 100 to 1. 円／ドル換算レートを100とすると，**千兆**が1兆の千倍だから，千兆円は10兆ドルと交換できる。@円（yen）とその略語¥は常に単数形

2) Function of organs　　臓器の機能

[1] The pancreas is the organ **responsible for** the breakdown of glucose.　　司る

[2] The pancreas **polices** the blood sugar level.　　管理する (i.e. to regulate)

[3] Exercise **encourages** the pancreas to secrete insulin.　　促す (i.e. to promote)
　　or　Insulin is the only hormone that **functions** in lowering the blood glucose level.

[4] The pancreas **releases** insulin into the bloodstream.　　分泌させる（i.e. to secrete）

[5] A measure of the hemoglobin bound to glucose over a period of time **provides a better overall picture** of glucose control than other measures.　　ある期間にわたり，血糖と結合したヘモグロビンを測定すると，値がばらつく他の指標よりも血糖値コントロールの**全体像をよく把握できる。**

[6] The liver **plays a major role in** metabolism of all three elemental nutrients, as well as synthesizes several kinds of protein compounds and detoxifies some poisonous substances.　　肝臓は三大栄養素（蛋白質，脂質，糖質：炭水化物）の代謝と，各種蛋白質の合成や，ある種の毒素の解毒に**重要な役割を果たす。**

[7] The kidneys **play an essential part in** maintaining **homeostasis**, by varying the amounts of substances leaving and entering the blood.　　腎臓は血管に流入・流失する物質量を変化させてホメオスタシス（恒常性）を保つ**本質的な役割を果たす**

3) Percentage or ratio　　割合

[1] The genetic factor **accounts for** only one-third of the risk factors.

②Of the risk factors, the rest **comprise** two thirds. 　分母は分子の単・複数に応じる
③It **consists of** three-quarters or less. 　　3 / 4以下
④It **constitutes** somewhere between 60 and 70 % 　60〜70%あたり
⑤The total naturally **amounts to** 100 percent. 　達する
⑥What percent does it account for? 　何%か？
　or　How large is the percentage?

Quiz

A. What hormone regulates the blood sugar level, and what happens if this hormone is insufficient?

B. What are the three causes of diabetes?

C. What does the doctor advise the patient to do for preventing diabetes?

D. What kind of sensation appears at the first stage of diabetes? Why?

E. What did Jack think aerobic exercise was, What is it actually?

F. What is basal metabolism?

Answers

A. Insulin. Surplus glycogen turns into fatty acid and is stored in the liver or in the subcutaneous layer as neutral fat.

B. Obesity, inactivity and aging

C. Exercise regularly and eat nutritious, balanced meals.

D. Thirst. This is because a lot of glucose is excreted through the kidneys promoting urination.

E. Aerobic dance accompanied by music. It is actually a type of moderate exercise during which one can talk to another person.

F. It is the minimal energy needed to maintain life, the energy needed even while sleeping so that the heart and other organs keep functioning.

3. Hyperuricemia due to excessive drinking

――過度の飲酒による高尿酸血症

　Drinking a lot of alcohol not only damages the liver causing **fatty liver**[*1] and hepatitis, but can also lead to **pancreatitis**[*2] and **hyperuricemia**[*3] - a metabolic state occurring in people who have a high level of **uric acid (UA)** [*4] and **blood urine nitrogen (BUN)** [*5] - usually without showing any symptoms.

Gout, a disease resulting from excess drinking, is dormant in an estimated one out of ten adults over forty years old. Gout, literally translated, is known as "zephyr pain" because the pain is very severe and often accompanied by other **complications**[*6] such as aggravated gouty kidney, that can lead to chronic renal insufficiency and the need for **dialysis**[*7]. The acute pain is caused by an increase in uric acid. When it increases, it is deposited as **urate crystals**[*8] in and around the joints. Increased levels in the urine may lead to the formation of renal **urate calculi**[*9]. Uric acid is produced in a ratio of 6 to 7 in the body, with the rest coming from dietary intake. It is excreted through the urine and mucus. Both excess production and lower excretion of uric acid contribute to a higher BUN level. As uric acid is the end product of **purine metabolism**[*10], one should try to avoid eating foods that contain purine, as well as avoiding excess drinking and overly-vigorous exercise that is said to promote purine production in the body. Eating lots of vegetables helps keep the blood alkaline.

Notes: *1 脂肪肝, *2 膵炎, *3 高尿酸血症, *4 尿酸, *5 血中尿酸窒素, *6 合併症, *7 透析, *8 尿酸結晶（塩）, *9 腎結石, *10 プリン代謝

Dialogue

Situation 1: Jack is complaining about the severe pain from gout to Mike, the doctor, who is teaching Jack about what causes the disease and how to cope with it.
ジャックが通風の痛みを例の医師，マイクに訴えている。マイクはジャックに通風の原因と，どのように対処するかを教えている。

Jack: Why does gout give me such intense pain?

Mike: When urinate crystals scatter from a joint, leukocytes concentrate around the scattered crystals in the bursa in order to attack them as **foreign bodies**. This action causes the area to become inflamed resulting in **throbbing** pain. This action of the leukocytes is called **phagocytosis**.　尿酸結晶が関節から剥離すると，滑液包内に散乱した結晶の周りに白血球が集まり，結晶を**異物**として攻撃する／これにより，その部分が炎症を起こして**ズキズキ痛む**（脈動性の痛み）／白血球のこのような活動を**貪食作用**という

Jack: I have been on the alert for diabetes. Why have I developed this ailment?

Mike: Because of alcohol and obesity. You've always been a party king - the MC of every event, haven't you?

Jack: You know that a capable director of a sales department must play such a role.
有能な営業部長は芸能部長（Master of Ceremonies: MC）でもある

Chapter IV. Suggestions based on laboratory test results

Mike: **Let** your liver **take a break** at least a couple of days a week. The liver is a chemical factory where harmful substances are broken down and detoxified. In the process of breaking alcohol down into water and carbon dioxide, toxic **acetaldehyde** is generated as a byproduct. If the amount of alcohol consumed is small, the liver can detoxify it using the **concerned enzyme** γ-GTP. In this process, energy-rich **ATP** (adenosine triphosphate) is also consumed and **uric acid** is produced accordingly. High alcohol intake damages the liver causing **fatty liver**; and the so-called **silent organ** cannot help but give a warning to the system by showing elevated levels of γ-GTP in serum, an indicator of an **alcoholic liver**. 　週に2日ほど**休肝日**をとる／肝臓は有害物質を分解・解毒する化学工場である／アルコールを水と2酸化炭素に分解する過程で**アセトアルデヒド**が副産物として生成される／その量が少ないと肝臓は**解毒作用に関係する酵素**、ガンマ GTP でアセトアルデヒドを解毒する／この課程で化学反応に富んだ **ATP** も消費され、その量に応じて**尿酸**が生成される／アルコール摂取量が多いと肝臓は害されて**脂肪肝**となり、**沈黙の臓器**と呼ばれる肝臓もたまらずに、**アルコール肝**の指標である"血清中のガンマ GTP の値が高い"との警告を出す

Jack: This test chart shows exclamation marks, or **dire warnings**, not only for γ-GTP level, but also other test results (See **Table 1**). 　γ-GTPだけでなく、他の検査値の横に感嘆符"！"**が不吉な警告としてついている**（**Table 1** 参照）

Mike: Whenever liver cells (**hepatocytes**) are damaged, levels of the **transaminases**, AST (GOT) and ALT (GPT) increase. Both are enzymes that act as **catalysts** in helping to **synthesize** amino acid. These enzymes increase in the serum due to cellular damage allowing leakage of them into circulation (**released enzyme**). AST is found particularly in heart, liver, muscle and kidney tissue. Among the two, ALT is a more **specific indicator** of liver function. Serum activity increases in patients with infectious hepatitis and cirrhosis of the liver, and also in **obstructive jaundice**. 　肝細胞が損傷されると、AST（GOT），ALT（GPT）双方の**トランスアミナーゼ**の値が上る／これらはアミノ酸**合成**の**触媒**としてはたらく酵素である／細胞の損傷により、これらが血中に流入し血清濃度が上がる（**逸脱酵素**）／GOT は特に、心臓、筋肉、腎組織にみられる／ALT はほぼ肝機能**固有の指標**であり、肝炎、肝硬変、**閉塞性黄疸**でこの値が高くなる

Table 1 Example results of laboratory tests for Jack
Jackの検査値の結果例

The ratio of **albumin** (ALB) **to globulin** (A/G) indicates abnormal liver function when the value is low and total protein (TP) level is normal. Here, the unit (IU/L/37℃) indicates "International Unit per liter at 37degrees C[*1]".
アルブミン対グロブリン比

	Tests		Results	Reference	Unit
Transaminases for liver & adjacent organs	Total Protein	TP	7.7	6.7～8.3	g/dL
	Albumin	ALB	4.7	3.8～5.3	〃
	A/G	AG	1.6	1.1～2.0	—
	AST (GOT)	AST	28	10～40	IU/L/37℃
	ALT (GPT)	ALT	22	5～45	
	LDH	LDH	342	250～420	
	Al-P	ALP	247	90～270	
	γ-GTP	GTP	! 77	M80 以下 (F30)	
	Cholinesterase	CHE	6484	3000～7000	
Lipid, uric acids & electrolytes for urinary system	Serum Amylase	SAMY	124	55～175	mg/dL
	Blood Urea Nitrogen	BUN	! 24	8～23	
	Creatinine	CRE	! 1.3	M 0.8～1.3 F 0.6～1.1	
	Uric Acid	UA	! 8.2	M 3.8～7.5 F 2.4～5.8	
	Total Cholesterol	TCH	! 224	120～219	
	High Density Lipoprotein	HDL	56	M 40～70 F 45～75	
	Triglyceride	TG	146	30～149	
	Sodium	Na	140	135～145	mEg[*2]/L
	Potassium	K	! 5.5	3.5～5.0	
	Chloride	Cl	104	98～108	

＊1 摂氏37°，＊2 ミリグラム当量（P86関連・補足表現参照）

Jack: How do you determine my gout condition from an alcoholic liver?

Mike: When the GOT level exceeds that of GPT with increased γ-GTP, it **indicates possible** alcoholic liver disease. If the ratio of GOT to GPT is more than double, it is said to **be indicative of** liver cancer. 　ガンマGTPの値が高くて，GOTの値がGPTの値より高いとき（i.e. GOT＞GPT）はアルコール肝の**可能性が高い**／もし，GPTに対するGOTの比が2を超えると（i.e. GOT／GPT＞2），肝臓癌の**可能性が高い**と言われている

Jack: What about my case?

Mike: **As far as** the data **goes**, your liver shows no sign of being a malignant case, with LDH (lactate dehydrogenase) barely within the **reference range** and the **biliary system** showing a normal level of ALP (Alkaline phosphatase). It can be said that your gout was derived from an alcoholic liver. 　検査値に関する限り，肝臓には悪性のものはない／LDH（乳酸脱水素酵素）もかろうじて**基準範囲**内だし，ALPの値も正常なので**胆道系**にも異常はない

Jack: That's a **hollow consolation** to me **now that** I am going to die in pain. Why has this happened to me? Where is **God in all** this suffering? What are the **odds** of me developing such a condition?　いまの私には**空々しい慰め**にしか聞こえない／痛みで死にそう**なんだから**／神も仏もない／どのくらいの**可能性**

Mike: The number of gout **candidates**, or people with latent potential for developing the disease, is estimated to be one out of ten adults above 40-years old. However, more than 90% of victims are male. 　40歳以上の大人で通風**予備軍**は10人に1人と推定されている／その9割以上が男性

Jack: It's not fair, is it?

Mike: **As is the case of** osteoporosis increasing mainly among females. The female hormone (estrogen) is associated with this trend. In this case, estrogen **counteracts** uric acid. 　骨粗鬆症が女性に多いの**と同様に**／女性ホルモンは通風発症の傾向に関係している／この場合は尿酸に対して**抑制効果**を持つ

Jack: Who is more likely to get gout?

Mike: It's more likely to be an obese person who is very sensitive to stress. Any person whose uric acid (UA) level exceeds 7.0/dl falls into the candidate group. The level of your UA is 8.2. **No wonder you are suffering** a gout attack. If you don't rectify the situation, you may develop a gouty kidney. In the worst case, it leads to dialysis. 　この値だと，**いつ通風発作が起き**

てもおかしくない

Jack: What do you mean by dialysis?

Mike: Dialysis is an artificial filtration system of waste materials from the blood and is used to replace failed kidney function. You need to have it done usually three times a week. Don't worry, though. This is your first attack. The **acute phase** doesn't last long - say about a week. In this phase, a **symptomatic treatment** is undergone using **antiphlogistic** that alleviates the pain. It serves to suppress that **phagocytosis**. As the medicine I'm giving you is associated with strong **side-effects**, take the tablet only once a day, never more. And **apply** this **cold pack** three times a day.　急性期は長くは続かない，1週間以内というところ／この期間には痛みを和らげる対処療法（palliative treatment）として抗炎症薬が使われる／これは白血球の貪食作用を抑制する／この種の薬は強い副作用がある／冷湿布を日に3度貼る

Jack: If the pain goes away, is it the end of this disease?

Mike: Oh, no! You still need **radical treatment** even after the pain has subsided, which is the **resting stage**. This disease behaves much like a dormant volcano; and **who knows** when it may erupt again.　痛みがとれたら根本療法が必要になる／痛みが治まっても，それは休止期である／ちょうど休火山のように，いつ噴火してもおかしくない

Jack: You're trying to frighten me again. A **scary scenario** is sure to follow as usual.　いつものように恐ろしい筋書がきっと続く

Mike: If you want to live free from pain all the way to your grave, take this medicine after the pain has gone. It should reduce the UA level to below five within two weeks. If so, I'll wait and see if the value stays low without the tablets for another two weeks. They say, "**The burnt child dreads the fire.**" But also they say, "**Once on shore, we pray no more.**" If you let the disease become chronic, or move **inward to the inveterate phase**, you'll **be associated with this medicine** to the grave to be sure. Such a case results from bad **compliance**.　羹（あつもの）に懲りてなますを吹く／咽もと過ぎれば熱さを忘れる／慢性化させて陳旧期まで長引かせると本当に死ぬまで薬づけになる／そうなるのはコンプライアンス（順守）が悪いから

Quiz

A. What is made as a byproduct in the process of alcohol being broken down into water and carbon dioxide?

B. Why did Mike tell Jack to let his liver take a break looking at the lab results?

C. What enzymes help synthesize amino acid as catalysts?

D. Which enzyme is a more specific indicator of liver function, AST (GOT) or ALT (GPT)?

E. Do Jack's test results indicate possible liver cancer? Why or why not?

F. Why did Mike make a decisive diagnosis of gout for Jack?

G. Why are women much less likely to suffer from gout?

H. Is his kidney damaged so severely that he has to have dialysis?

I. Why is chronic gout called a disease of bad compliance?

J. Roughly estimate the LDL level for Jack by the method described earlier.

Answers

A. Acetaldehyde.

B. The level of γ-GTP was abnormally high.

C. The transaminases AST (GOT) and ALT (GPT).

D. ALT

E. No, because the ratio of GOT to GPT is less than double. In addition, both of the levels of LDH and ALP are within the reference range.

F. The level of his uric acid (UA) was as high as 8.2.

G. The female hormone (estrogen) counteracts uric acid.

H. No. His level of BUN* marginally exceeds the reference level.

　＊blood urea nitrogen：血中尿素窒素

I. A victim acts like "a child burnt by fire" just after severe pain; but tends to neglect taking medicine regularly during the dormant phase of the disease - as the saying goes, "Once on shore, we pray no more."

J. 139

Situation 2: Jack goes to get a shot and asks Karen, a nurse whom he knows well, about blood and urine tests.　ジャックは注射を打ちに行き，なじみの看護師，カレンに血液検査と尿検査について尋ねる。

Karen:　**Roll up** your sleeve **to** the elbow, please. Could you place your arm here? I need your arm fully extended with your palm up. Make a fist and **clench** it tight.　肘まで袖を**捲り上げる**／げんこつをしっかり**握り締める**

Jack:　I always feel sorry to see a nurse at a loss to find a puncture site. The rub-

	ber tube strapped around my big arm usually doesn't work to make the veins **stand out**.　腕に巻いたゴムチューブは，丸太のような腕から血管を**浮き出さす**ことができない
Karen:	I'll manage fine. Stay still with your mouth **zipped**, please.　喋らないで
Jack:	It didn't hurt at all. Only a **prick** as if a mosquito bit me.　ちっとも痛くない／蚊が**ちくり**と刺したよう
Karen:	Don't bend your arm or take off the tape until the bleeding stops.
Jack:	What will you test with this blood?
Karen:	Uric acid, BUN and Creatinine (CRE) levels among other things that are indicators of kidney (renal) function and enzyme release from the liver.
Jack:	Mike only told me about liver (hepatic) function, mentioning the strong or **strained connection** of alcohol and liver stress.　アルコールとの関係にこじつけて
Karen:	I think he explained to you causes of gout. Kidney damage is a **product** of the disease **by and large**. Many people, 40 percent in fact, have an overactive carbohydrate metabolism and overproduce purine, the end product.　腎障害は**大体**において痛風の**結果**である
Jack:	Then, I might have gotten gout from kidney malfunction, not from fatty liver due to alcohol and obesity.
Karen:	Purine is broken down into waste at the liver by an enzyme and then circulates in the bloodstream until it is excreted as urine or stool. Usually production and excretion levels are balanced. Uric acid increases in the blood if the kidney doesn't filtrate the waste sufficiently, or if there is an overproduction of purine in the body.
Jack:	It's like the question of **which came first**, the chicken or the egg?　鶏と卵ではどちらが先にできたかという問題と同じ
Karen:	Uric acid increases due to excess drinking and or obesity.
Jack:	Oh, you're **sounding like** Bob.　マイクと同じことを**言って責める**
Karen:	Anyway, take this cup and fill it one third with urine. Then, take it to the lab for urine tests (**urinalysis**), being sure to label it with your name.　このコップに名前を貼って**尿検査室**に持っていく
Jack:	Why a urine test in addition to the blood test?
Karen:	When it comes to kidney function, a blood test alone is not accurate enough for evaluation. Both CRE and BUN don't decrease until the kidney function

is lowered by one-third the normal level. On the contrary, urine tests can find the presence of protein or red cells in the urine. A healthy kidney won't allow blood cells or protein larger than **albumin** to pass through the barrier. Even if these substances have once passed the **glomerulus**, all of these important substances are reabsorbed into the blood through the **uriniferous tubule**. If red blood cells exist, it indicates the possible presence of **urate calculi**. When protein is found in the urine, it indicates that there may be something wrong in the glomerulus. You can see bead-like bubbles in the urine if protein exists in it (**proteinuria**). But exceptions sometimes occur so that one must **rule them out** by further examination (**Fig.3**).　アルブミン（単純蛋白）／糸球体／尿細管／尿路結石／蛋白尿／除外する

Jack:　　What a complicated explanation.

Karen:　　The kidneys are located close to the back, the right one lower than the left one due to **pressure from the liver above**. Let's compare the kidney with an egg. The **cortex** is **eggwhite**, so to speak, and the analogous part of the **medulla** in which the **renal pelvis** is connected to the ureter is the **yolk**. In the cortex, there are many **clusters of calipers** (**glomerulus**), and an important part consists of a **nephron** unit along with fine ureters (**tubles**). Urine secreted by millions of nephrons collects in the renal pelvis before entering the ureter. Repeating secretion and reabsorption, 10 percent of uric acid is finally secreted in the urine. When the UA level is high, it starts to crystallize, damaging the **collecting system** and causing an abnormality. This is what I mean by the relationship of the chicken and the egg.　肝臓による**上からの圧迫**／皮質：白身／髄質：黄身／腎盂／毛細管の房（糸球体）／ネフロン／尿細管／尿路系

Jack:　　Mike recommended me (to)* take a lot of vegetables and milk. Why is that?

Karen:　　They change the urine from an acidic condition to alkaline, which promotes the secretion of uric acid.

Jack:　　Do you dip a strip of paper into the urine to determine the pH by color?

Karen:　　Yes, when we are in a hurry. If you want more information about it, ask a **medical technologist** (MT) about the **qualitative analysis** of **hydrogen ion exponent** using a special instrument. Don't forget to collect the **mid-stream**

＊recommendに続く動詞は原形となるが，米口語では（to）を使う場合が多い。

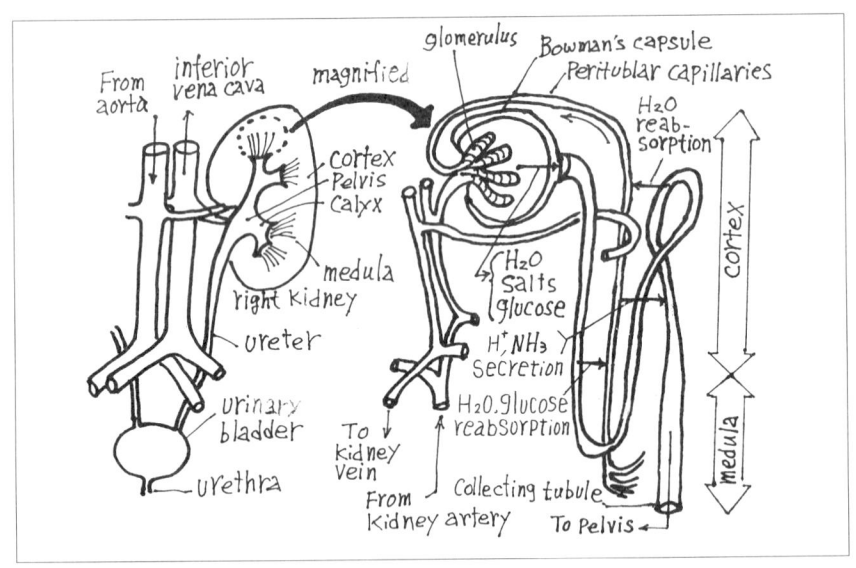

Fig. 3 Posterior view of right kidney (left), and magnified nephron unit and uriniferous tubes (right).
The medulla contains millions of microscopic units called nephrons that are functional units of the kidneys. Urine is formed in the nephrons by the process of filtration, and repeating reabsorption and secretion occur between peritubular capillaries and the collecting tubule. Glomeruli in the Bowman's capsule consist of a cluster of capillaries which are important parts of each nephron. The urine secreted by the nephrons collects through the collecting tubes in the renal pelvis before entering the ureters.

	urine.　臨床検査技師／定量測定／水素イオン指数＝pH（ピーエイチ）／中間尿
Jack:	I'm not good at it. Once it starts flowing, it **won't** stop. Do you have any **tips**?　いったん出始めるとどうにも止まらない／いい**コツ**がないか
Karen:	You just have to try as firmly as possible to shutoff the flow.
Jack:	You're talking about **number 1** now, not **number 2**.　排便でなく排尿の問題のはず
Karen:	The **figure-eight shaped** muscle (pelvic-floor muscle) at the bottom is composed of two circles that move together, the front circle closing the urethra and the rear circle closing the anus. Elderly persons tend to have a loose pelvic muscle that often leads to **incontinence of urine**. But the back muscle part works firmly enough even for the urethra if you **hold** your stomach

in. お尻の**八の字型の**筋肉（骨盤底筋）は同時に動く2つの輪があって，前の輪で尿道を，後ろの輪で肛門を絞める／老齢者のこの筋肉は緩みがちでときどき**尿失禁**を引き起こす／お腹を**引っ込ませる**と後ろの輪が前の輪までしっかりと閉じる

Jack: I got it. It's the **same as** when we try to stop **flatulence** from coming out. 出かかった**おなら**（breaking wind）を止めるときの**要領**だね

Karen: I see. さあね（軽く受け流す）

Quiz

A. How does Jack ask Karen about his disease?

B. What is Karen's answer?

C. Why is a blood test only not enough for the evaluation of kidney function?

D. What can a urine test show concerning kidney function?

E. When protein is found in the urine, what part of the kidney is malfunctioning?

Answers

A. He makes an excuse connecting his disease with kidney function.

B. Overall, uric acid increases by excess drinking and/or obesity.

C. Because both CRE and BUN don't decrease until kidney function is as low as one-third the normal level.

D. Protein or red cells

E. Glomerulus

Relevant expressions and additional phrases

1) Absence　　休暇

①She is taking sick leave.　病欠中である

　　cf. This vending machine is taking "sick leave."　この自販機は"病欠中"（故障中）です。

②She is taking maternity leave.　産休中である

③She is on monthly leave.　生理休暇中である

④He is AWOL (Absent Without Leave) today again.　今日も無断欠勤（ずる休み）である

⑤A **truant** is someone who is absent from work without notice or explanation.　無断欠席者

2) Limit of patience　　我慢の限界
1. **I can't stand for** (put up with) his treatment any longer.　　もう我慢ができない
2. The patient **is fed up with** the severe pain, but is **complying less with** the doctor's advice as time goes on.　　余りの痛さにうんざりするが，時が経つにつれて医師の指示に従わなくなる
3. This is the last straw.　　これが我慢の限界

3) Resignation　　諦め（しかたがない）
1. I can't help but wait and see for the time being.　　しばらく様子をみるより～
2. It can't be helped but to wait and see.　　待つしかない
3. We have no choice but to follow the trend.　　流れに任せるしか～
4. There is no other way but to take it as it comes.　　なるようにしかならない
5. If it happens, it happens.　　なればなったとき

4) Know-how　　コツ（秘策）
1. Please, show me your techniques and tips.　　技術のコツ
2. Tell me the secret (or trick).　　秘策
3. He'll soon have a knack for it.　　要領をつかむ
4. After much trial and error, he'll know the ropes.　　コツを知る
5. He got the hang of it.　　コツを掴んだ

5) Common expressions of excretion　　排泄の一般表現
1. empty one's bladder (do number one) →urinate　　排尿する
2. relieve yourself (do number two) →evacuate　　排便をする
3. have loose bowels →have diarrhea　　下痢をする
4. have no bowel movement→ have constipation　　便秘をする
5. wet one's pants→have incontinence of urine　　失禁する

6) Proverbs / sayings　　諺・格言
1. It is easier said than done.　　言うはやすし，行うは難し
   cf. That's not the way things go.　　そうは問屋が卸さない
2. A cold may develop into all kinds of illnesses.　　風邪は万病の元
3. Sound body, sound mind.　　健全な身体に健全な精神が宿る
   cf. The converse is also true.　　逆もまた真なり

④Out of sight, out of mind. 　去るもの，日々に疎し
⑤The mind rules the body. 　病は気から
⑥Too much is as bad as too little. 　過ぎたるは及ばざるがごとし
⑦Prevention is better than cure. 　転ばぬ先の杖
⑧A little knowledge is a dangerous thing. 　生兵法は怪我のもと
⑨The burnt child dreads the fire. 　羹（あつもの）に懲りてなますを吹く
⑩Once on shore, we pray no more. 　喉元過ぎれば熱さを忘れる
⑪Where there's a will there's a way. 　継続は力なり

Exercise IV.

IV.-1. Translate Japanese into English referring to the technical terms below.

coronary heart disease：冠動脈疾患，so called "good cholesterol"：善玉コレステロール，動脈硬化：arterial sclerosis

冠動脈疾患へのHDLの役割は要因よりも防御にある。なぜなら，HDLは余剰のコレステロールと結合しそれを肝臓へ送り，そこで余剰のコレステロールは代謝され血流から除去されるからである。それが故に，動脈硬化の最大要因となるLDLと異なり，HDLは善玉コレステロールと呼ばれる。

IV.-2. Translate English into Japanese referring to the technical terms below.

fluid balance：体液平衡，dehydration：脱水症，overhydration:：過水症，electrolyte：電解質，chloride：クロル，homeostasis：恒常性，acid-base balance：酸塩基平衡，body fluid：体液，distal tubule：尿細管

A normal human body maintains a **fluid balance** known as homeostasis for all components. For example, the total volume of water is maintained, on the most part, by adjusting water intake to the output level of urine. A fluid imbalance causes **dehydration** or **overhydration**, yet causes an increase in blood concentration of **electrolytes**. Electrolytes are compounds that dissociate in solution to yield positively charged particles or cations and negatively charged particles, anions, such as chloride (Cl^-). Important cations include sodium (Na^+), calcium (Ca^{++}) and potassium (K^+), etc. Since the kidney acts as the chief regulator of these electrolytes, an imbalance can indicate kidney malfunction. Another health indicator role for the kidney is to regulate the **acid-base balance** of **body fluids**. The indicator is a given fluid's hydrogen-ion concentration or pH. More specifically, a pH of 7.0 is normal or neutral in reaction, neither acid nor alkaline. The kidneys are vital organs that maintain homeostasis of pH. The **distal tubules** of the kidneys rid the blood of excess acid and conserve the acid balance. Notice that urine pH is more acidic - one to two notches lower than the pH of blood at 7- because of the urine becomes acidic before discharge.

IV.-3. Answer the following question in English using the key words below.

Question: What is your advice in keeping oneself free of lifestyle disease?

obesity：肥満症, hyperlipidemia：高脂血症, arterial sclerosis：動脈硬化, health supplements：代替栄養補助食品, aerobic exercise：有酸素運動

Example answerは巻末（付録の前）に掲載

Chapter V.

Musculoskeletal Injuries
筋骨格損傷

Skeletal injuries (fractures) are potentially serious since not only is the skeleton injured but also the soft tissue in the immediate surrounding area. **Tendons**[*1], **ligaments**[*2] muscles, nerves, blood vessels and skin may also be involved. Muscle is usually attached to bone by tendon through which the mechanism of muscle contraction is carried out. All joints are surrounded by a **joint capsule**[*3] lined by membrane which is strengthened and protected by bands of connective tissue (ligaments). Ligaments limit and maintain abnormal movement of the joint (**passive stability**) [*4] made by muscle activity (**active stability**) [*5]. Skeletal fractures may be classified as **transverse, oblique, spiral** or **comminuted**[*6]. When the fractured ends of the bone pierce the skin, the injury is known as an **open** or **compound fracture**[*7]. With compound fractures there is a great risk of infection of the bone, and special treatment is required. If a bone attached to a muscle or ligament has been torn away, it is called an **avulsion fracture**[*8].

The different types of disorder due to trauma are **dislocations**[*9] of joints with or without joint ligament injuries. For a dislocation to occur, at least part of the capsule and its ligaments must be torn. Therefore, any dislocation involves injuries to these structures and sometimes to articular cartilage. **Total dislocation (luxation)** [*10] of a joint indicates the opposing surfaces have become separated and are no longer in contact with each other. **Partial dislocation (subluxation)** [*11] of a joint indicates that the articular surfaces remain in partial contact with each other but no longer correctly aligned. Again, there may be capsule, ligament and cartilage injuries. Disruption of the fibers of the ligament is often accompanied by bleeding which spreads into surrounding tissues and is frequently seen as **bruising**[*12].

Exercises for a successful rehabilitation program after a musculoskeletal injury should

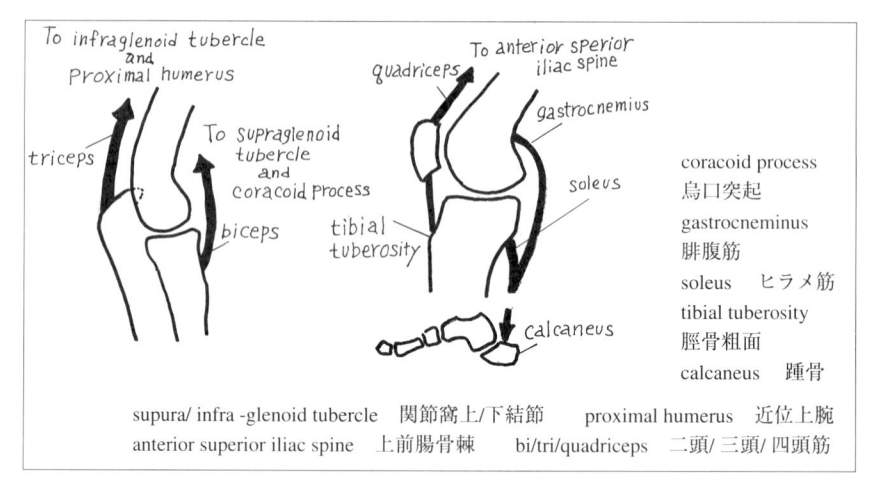

Fig. 1 Antagonism of joint muscles of elbow (left) and knee (right)
肘（左）と膝（右）関節筋の拮抗作用

Figure labels:
- To infraglenoid tubercle and Proximal humerus — triceps
- To supraglenoid tubercle and coracoid Process — biceps
- tibial tuberosity
- To anterior superior iliac spine — quadriceps
- gastrocnemius
- soleus
- calcaneus

coracoid process　烏口突起
gastrocneminus　腓腹筋
soleus　ヒラメ筋
tibial tuberosity　脛骨粗面
calcaneus　踵骨
supura/infra-glenoid tubercle　関節窩上/下結節　proximal humerus　近位上腕
anterior superior iliac spine　上前腸骨棘　bi/tri/quadriceps　二頭/三頭/四頭筋

aim to expand **range of motion** (passive and active ROM) [13] and preserve the **strength** [14], **elasticity and contractility** [15] of the **joint components** [16]. There are three types of contraction as follows: the **isometric** (or static) **work** [17] contraction which includes contractions without a change in muscle length; the **concentric contraction** [18] in which muscles contract and shorten in length simultaneously so that the attachments are drawn closer together, as is the case with **bicep muscles** [19] when the arm is bent (at the same time, **tricep muscles** [20] extend **antagonistically** [21]) (**Fig. 1**) ; and the **eccentric contraction** [22] where muscles contract and lengthen simultaneously so their attachments are drawn apart for maintaining the same length (like the contraction of the **quadriceps muscles** [23], for example, which function in both joint movement and stabilization when walking downstairs). Diagnosis and treatment of injuries should be undergone after a preliminary x-ray examination in order to ensure if a fracture is present or not and to monitor **interval changes** [24] of the healing process.

Notes: ＊1 腱，＊2 靭帯，＊3 関節包，＊4 他動的安定性，＊5 自動的（随意的）安定性，＊6 （横，斜，らせん，粉砕）骨折，＊7 開放骨折，＊8 剥離骨折，＊9 脱臼，＊10 完全脱臼，＊11 亜脱臼，＊12 打撲傷，＊13 関節可動域，＊14 筋力，＊15 弾性と収縮性，＊16 関節構成要素（骨・筋等の軟部組織），＊17 等尺性作用，＊18 求心性収縮，＊19 二頭筋，＊20 三頭筋，＊21 拮抗作用として，＊22 遠心性収縮，＊23 四頭筋，＊24 経時変化

Chapter V. Musculoskeletal Injuries 111

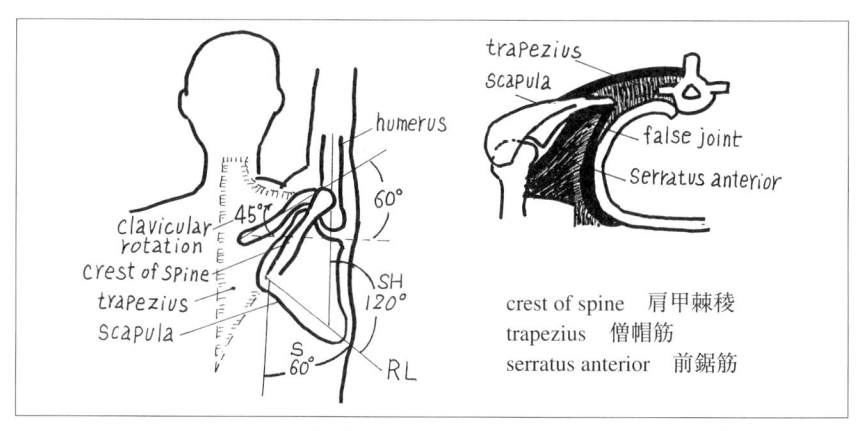

Fig. 2 Scapulohumeral rhythm (left) and false joint of shoulder girdle (right).
肩甲上腕リズム（左）と肩甲‐胸郭仮性関節（右）。上腕骨の挙上に伴い肩甲骨が回旋する。正常な肩甲上腕関節では、肩甲骨内縁線（RL）が矢状面となす角を1とすると，上腕骨・内縁線間の角度（SH）は2となる。図のような上腕最大挙上では60°：120°，また，水平外転では30°：60°となる。

1. Shoulder girdle injuries ——肩帯損傷

A. Dislocation and subluxation of the shoulder joint
——肩関節の脱臼と亜脱臼

The shoulder girdle is formed by the clavicle which is articulated with the sternum in the medial and scapula in the lateral; the side of the scapula is also articulated with the proximal portion of the humerus forming the **gleno-humeral joint**[*1]. The shoulder girdle is very complex both in its arrangement and number of component parts. When raising one's arm, first the **deltoid muscle**[*2] starts to lift up the humerus, then the scapula tilts and the **supraspinatus muscle**[*3] swings the arm from the side, finally the crank-like claviclar shaft which is concave on the downward side **turns upside down**[*4] to complete the **abduction**[*5]. The shoulder girdle joints make a contribution to nearly every movement that takes place in this region (**scapulohumeral rhythm**[*6]). This is particularly true of movements of scapulae which **compensate**[*7] the limited mobility of the gleno-humeral joint (**Fig. 2**).

There are two types of dislocation: one is **traumatic dislocation**[*8] mainly caused by

```
Subscapularis.m (SSC)    Hill-Sachs lesion    deltoid muscle    acromion
                         Bankart lesion                          coracoid process
    supraspinatus.m                              SSP          AN
      (SSP)                                                   GT
    infraspinatus.m                                           BG      GHJ
      (ISP)            glenoid labrum           SSC           LT
    teres minor muscle                          ISP
```

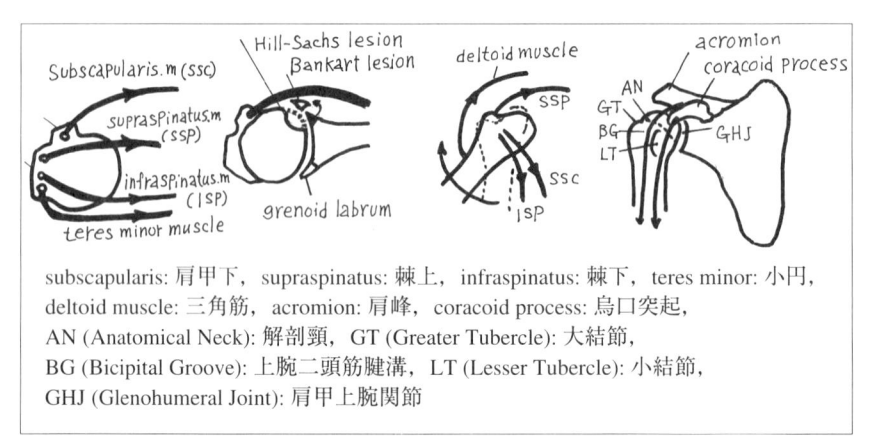

subscapularis: 肩甲下， suprapinatus: 棘上， infraspinatus: 棘下， teres minor: 小円，
deltoid muscle: 三角筋， acromion: 肩峰， coracoid process: 烏口突起，
AN (Anatomical Neck): 解剖頸， GT (Greater Tubercle): 大結節，
BG (Bicipital Groove): 上腕二頭筋腱溝， LT (Lesser Tubercle): 小結節，
GHJ (Glenohumeral Joint): 肩甲上腕関節

Fig. 3 Shoulder cuffs　肩腱板

a violent force directly applied to the shoulder (except for a few cases indirectly due to a fall on the outstretched hand). Such dislocations are frequently associated with fractures of the neck of humerus (**surgical neck**) *[9] and of avulusion fractures of the **greater tubercle** (tuberosity) *[10], the site of **insertion***[11] of the supraspinatus muscle or of the **lesser tubercle** (**subscapularis insertion site**) *[12]. The other type of dislocation is **recurrent subluxation***[13] caused by an **unstable shoulder joint***[14] that slips backward or forward although dislocation is not total. A **glenoid labrum***[15] tear is commonly associated with anterior dislocation and subluxation of the shoulder or with **a generative lesion** *[16]. The generative **shoulder cuffs***[17] **are subject to tearing** *[18] and often a cause of **frozen shoulder***[19] or restriction of shoulder movement due to pain (**Fig. 3**).

An x-ray examination can confirm a diagnosis by showing skeletal changes along the anterior edge of the joint socket (**glenoid cavity***[20]). Such an exam will also help verify or **rule out***[21] the presence of a fracture. Rehabilitation starts after 2-6 weeks with early range of motion and strength training, especially overhead rotation exercises.

Notes: *1 肩甲上腕関節， *2 三角筋， *3 棘上筋， *4 ひっくり返る， *5 外転，
　　　*6 肩甲上腕リズム， *7 代償する， *8 外傷性脱臼， *9 外科頸， *10 大結節， *11 起始部， *12 小結節（肩甲下筋の起始部）， *13 習慣性脱臼， *14 動揺性肩関節， *15 関節唇， *16 退行性病変， *17 肩腱板， *18 断裂しやすい， *19 五十肩， *20 関節窩， *21 （要因を）除外する

Chapter V. Musculoskeletal Injuries   113

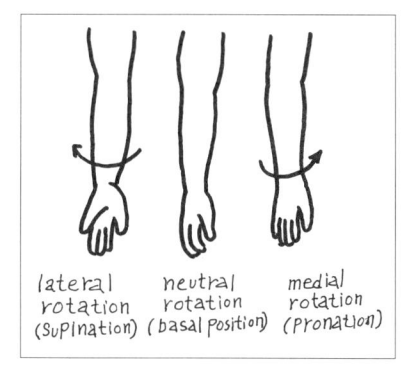

Fig. 4 Forearm motions and positions
前腕の運動と位置
supination　回外
basal positioning　基本肢位
pronation　回内

lateral rotation (supination)　neutral rotation (basal position)　medial rotation (pronation)

B. Dislocation of the acromiocravicular joint

——肩鎖関節脱臼

1) Patient's complaints　　患者の愁訴

1. I feel pain in my shoulder when I raise my arm higher than the shoulder.　　腕を肩より高くすると
2. I feel a **click or locking** when I raise and rotate my arm (overhead abduction and rotation).　　ひっかかり（嵌頓）／（挙上外転・回転）
3. I feel pain when I press the swollen part (**tenderness**).　　腫れた部分を押すと痛みを感じる（**圧痛**）。

2) Radiographic examinations　　X線検査

a) Anteroposterior projection (AP)　　前後方向撮影

1. Put your **back** against the cassette.　　カセッテに**背**をつける
2. Turn your palm so it faces **out** [so the greater tubercle position is profiled on the lateral aspect of the humerus (external rotation position: 外旋位)] (**Fig. 4**).　　掌が**表**を向くように
3. Rest the palm of your right hand against your thigh (neutral rotation position: 中間位).　　"気をつけ"の手の位置
4. Bend your arm a little and put the back of your hand on your hip [so the lesser tubercle position is profiled pointing medially (internal rotation position: 内旋位)].　　手の甲を腰につる

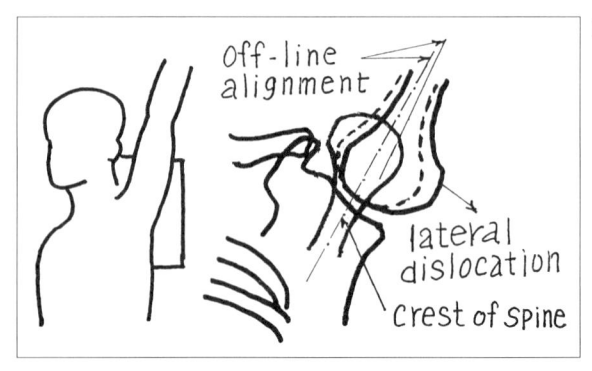

Fig. 5 Zero-position 前後最大挙上位
off-line alignment 偏位（スリッピング）
lateral dislocation 側方脱臼
crest of spine (of scapula) 肩甲棘稜

b) Weight-bearing position　　荷重位

1. Let's take additional x-rays holding weights in each hand for checking if dislocation or subluxation is present.　　今度は錘を持って
2. If the ligaments and the joint capsule tear, the joint will be wider on the separated side.

c) AP projection with the upper arm abducted upward　　前後方向挙上位

(1) **Upright zeroposition**[*1]　立位ゼロポジション (Active-abducted arm: 自立外転)

1. Raise the arm as high as comfortably possible and hold it steady at that position [a position where **shoulder cuffs are at rest,** which allows us to observe posterior **slipping** of the **humeral head** from the glenoid cavity, showing an off-line position with the **crest of spine**] (**Fig. 5**).　　すべての**肩腱板**が**安静位**である／すべり症／上腕骨骨頭／肩甲棘
2. Slowly **let the air out** and then stop breathing [Respiration is suspended at the end of exhalation].　　息を吐き終わった後で呼吸を止める

(2) **Recumbent zeroposition**[*2]　臥位ゼロポジション (Passive-abducted: 他動的外転)

1. Lie on your back on the table.
2. Rest your palms at your sides.
3. Let me move your upper arm up to the correct position [so that the axis of the

---

[*1] 上腕肩挙上時の肩関節安定位で，Radiographyでは慣例的に最大挙上位と呼んでいるが，Kinesiologyからみれば立位のゼロ肢位撮影である。

[*2] 上肢中間位から上腕側方挙上（abduction）150°，水平屈曲（horizontal flexion / adduction：正中冠状面から前方へ）30°。

Fig. 6　　**Fig. 7**

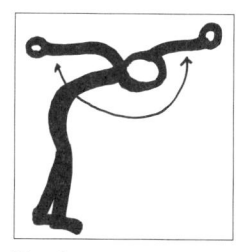

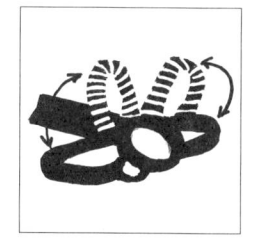

humerus is aligned parallel with the crest of scapular spine].

4 Tell me immediately if you feel pain in your shoulder.

3) **Rehabilitation**　　リハビリテーション

Mobility exercises　　可動運動

a) **Pendular movements**　　振り子運動

1 **Spread your feet apart** and lean your body forward (**Fig. 6**).　　両足を開いて前傾姿勢をとる

Swing the injured arm **forward** and **backward**.　　悪い方の腕を**前後**に振る

2 ～ **from side to** side in front of you.　　体の前で**左右**に振る

3 ～ in a circle, **clockwise** and **anti-clockwise** in turn.　　時計，反時計方向に交互に円を描く

b) **Scapula abduction and adduction**　　肩甲骨の外転と内転

1 Lie down **on your back** (in a supine position) and **clasp your hands** behind your head (**Fig. 7**).　　仰向きに寝て（仰臥位に），頭の後ろで**両手を組む**

Bring your arms **in** and **out in turn**.　　腕を広げたり狭めたり繰り返す

2 Stand up, now. Place your hands behind you.　　両手を背中に回す

Move your hands **as high up your back** as possible.　　できるだけ高く後ろ手を上げる

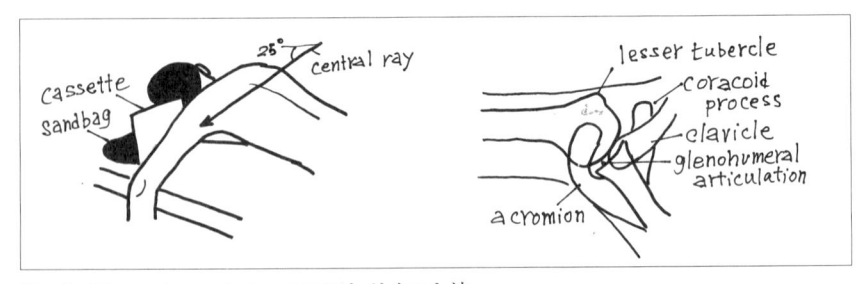

Fig. 8 West point method　ウエストポイント法

C.　Subluxation associated with glenoid labrum tear
　　　　　　　　　　　　　　　　——関節唇の剥離に伴う亜脱臼

1) Radiographic examinations
a) **Inferosuperior axial position (West Point Method)**　下・上方向軸位（ウエストポイント位）

　① Lie on the bed **on your stomach** (in a prone position) **(Fig. 8)**.　腹ばいに寝る（腹臥位に）

　② **Turn** your **face** the other way so your cheek rests on the pad (cf. **face** the other way).　顔をあちらに向ける（比較：**体全体を**あちらに向ける）

　③ **Extend** your arm (of affected side) **out** (abduct the arm 90 degrees).　悪いほうの手を横に出す（90°外転）

　④ Bend your arm so that the forearm **rests ove**r the edge of the table.　腕を曲げて前腕が寝台の**縁で垂れる**

　⑤ Don't move so the film (cassette) **will not shift its position against your shoulder**, since it's supported only by the pressure from a sandbag.　フィルム（カセット）は砂袋の圧力だけで**肩に寄りかかっている**だけだから

　⑥ You don't need to take a deep breath during x-rays; just hold your breath to **stay really still**.　ただ動かないために息を止めているだけ

b) **Stryker Notch Method**　ストライカー撮影法

　① Lie on your back with your right hand on top of your head **(Fig. 9)**.

　② Direct your elbow vertically keeping the upper arm parallel with the body (sagittal plane).

　③ The x-ray beam is directed at your armpit (30 degrees cephalic), so be sure not to

Chapter V. Musculoskeletal Injuries 117

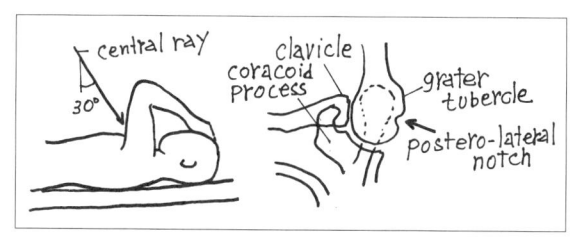

Fig. 9 Stryker notch method　ストライカー法

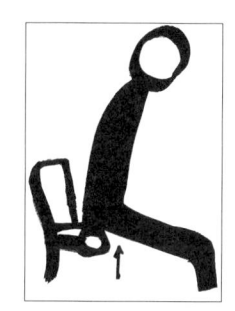

Fig. 10

move your arm.

3) Rehabilitation
a) Strength exercises　筋力運動
1. Sit **in** a chair.　（肘当てがなければ on a table）
2. Do **press-ups** by lifting your upper body with your arms (**Fig. 10**).　腕の力で上半身を**浮かせる**
3. Lie down on your stomach on the floor.
4. Do press-ups on the floor **facing down**. Extend and hold your arms **at full length** for several seconds.　うつ伏せで／腕をいっぱいに伸ばして
5. Don't confuse them with **push-ups**.　腕立て伏せと勘違いしないで

b) Static stretching exercises　ストレッチ
1. Hold your arms **straight out in front** of your body and press your hands together with increasing resistance[for **spinators** of the arm].　腕をまっすぐ前にのばして／両手の押し合う力を増して／腕の**外転筋群**の強化（**Fig. 3** 参照）
2. Next, bend your elbows and **press your hands together** for several seconds.　両肘を張ったまま，**両手に力を入れる**（念仏の姿勢で）
3. Stand **in front of an open door way** and put a hand on each side of the door frame.
4. Then, stretch by twisting your body to the left and right in turn so the **respective** arm and shoulder rotate outward [for **abductors** and **medial rotators** of the upper arm as well as **extensors** of the elbow] (**Fig. 11**).　開いたドアの入り口の前に立ち／ストレッチをしている側の腕と肩が前転するように［上腕の**外転筋群**と**内旋筋群**および肘の**伸展筋群**の強化］

Quiz

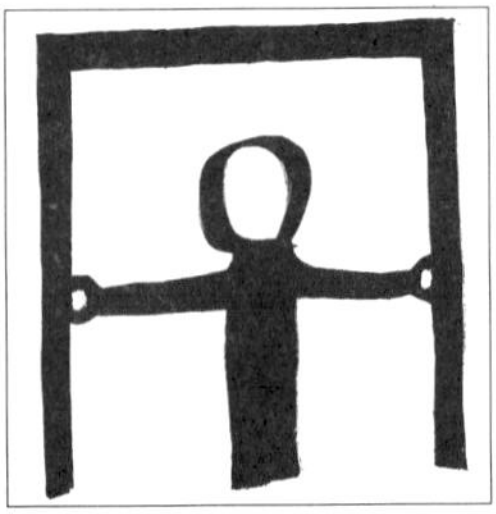

A. What muscles are involved in the rotator cuff; and where are their names derived from? Answer the questions looking at **Fig. 3**, if necessary.

B. Why is the scapula much more flexible in movements than other joint movements? List the four kinds of movement in combination with the respective muscles.

Fig. 11

C. Why does recurrent dislocation occur for a person who has experienced a glenoid labrum tear?

D. Choose the correct answer in the parentheses.
When standing in the anatomical position and the arm is flexed, the humerus rotates (medially / laterally) because of relaxation of the biceps. When the arm is fully elevated in the **fundamental position**, the S-shaped clavicle turns the inner curvature concave (inferiorly / superiorly) to adjust its length in scapulohumeral rhythm.
基本肢位（上肢の中間位）（**Fig. 41** 参照）

E. Choose the correct answer in the parentheses.
The **acromion** is the projection of the scapula extending (over / under) the humerus towards the upper (anterior / posterior) aspect of the scapula. The **coracoid process** is a beak-like process of the scapula projected (anteriorly / posteriorly) and to the (medial / lateral) side of the head of the humerus.　肩峰／烏口突起（**Fig. 3** 参照）

Answers

A. The **supraspinatus** acts as an abductor, **infraspinatus** acts as a **lateral rotator**, **teres minor** works as an adductor and lateral rotator, and **subscapularis** as a medial rotator.

B. Scapulae form **false joints** which allow them linear movement over the underlying rib cage with help from the **serratus muscle** and **trapezius muscle** for **protraction / retraction** (or rotating around chest laterally or medially) in addition to elevation and depression. These two **antagonistic muscles** can also allow angular motion by combining **upward / downward movement** and **abduction / adduction**.　仮性関節／前鋸筋／僧帽筋／（前突 / 後退）／拮抗筋（挙上 / 下制運動）／（外転 / 内転，または上方 / 下方回旋）

C. The glenohumeral joint is a **ball-and socket joint**. The socket (glenoid cavity) is shallow but deepened by a surrounding wall of **fibrocartilage** or glenoid labrum. If a part of the labrum tears, and a fracture exists in a part of the ball of the humeral head, especially in the posterolateral part (Hill-Sachs impression fracture*), recurrent dislocation occurs when the defected parts meet with the arm abducted and spinated together.　球関節 (P138参照) ／線維軟骨／ ＊上腕骨頭後外側部の骨欠損

D. medially, superiorly

E. over, posterior, anteriorly, medial

2. Elbow injuries　　　　　　　　　　　　　　　——肘の損傷

The elbow joint consists of three bones. On the distal humerus, the **trochlea**[1] articulates with the **trochlea notch**[2] of the ulna and **capitulum**[3] articulates with the head of the radius (**radial head**[4]). When flexing the arm, the **coronoid process**[5] **tucks into**[6] the **coronoid fossa**[7] and at full extension of the arm, the **olecranon process**[8] fits in the **olecranon fossa**[9]. When the arm is rotating medially (in **pronation**[10]), the radius turns (**radiates**[11]) and crosses over the ulna at its upper third. Because of this, a muscle must be attached to the radius to have an effect of pronation or **spination**[12]. At the anterior arm, the **biceps brachii muscle**[13], simply called biceps, crosses the elbow joint on the **radial tuberosity**[14]. Because it spans the elbow joint anteriorly and obliquely, it functions as a good elbow **flexor**[15] and **spinator**[16]. The strongest flexor is the **brachial muscle**[17] because it isn't attached to the radius, therefore, it specializes in flexion. The **triceps muscle**[18] makes up the entire muscle mass of the posterior arm. Different from the biceps, it spans the elbow vertically. It is very effective in elbow extension but can play no role in arm rotation because it isn't attached to the radius (See **Fig. 1**).

In the **anatomical position**[19], the longitudinal axis of the humerus and forearm forms an angle called the **caring angle**[20]. Thanks to this angle, the hand can rotate inside and the forearm can be aligned with that of the upper arm during elbow flexion. This helps get one's hand to the mouth (**Fig. 12**).

Notes:　＊1 滑車，＊2 滑車切痕，＊3 小頭，＊4 橈骨頭，＊5 鉤状突起，＊6 嵌頓，＊7 鉤状窩，＊8 肘頭突起，＊9 肘頭窩，＊10 回内，＊11 放射状に広がる，＊12 回外，＊13 二頭（腕頭骨）筋〔単に biceps (muscle) ともいう〕，＊14 橈骨結節，＊15 回内筋，＊16 回外筋，＊17 腕橈骨筋，＊18 （上腕）三頭筋，

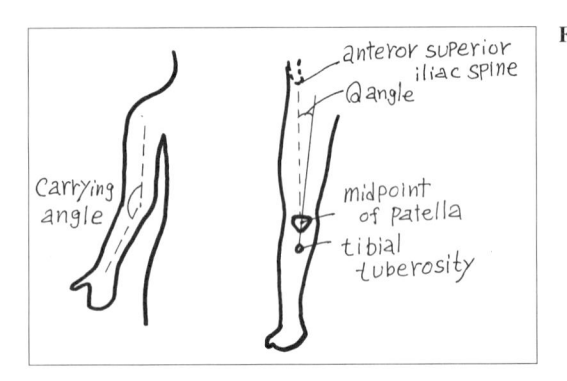

Fig. 12 Carrying angle and Q angle
肘角とQ角

＊19 解剖学的正面（肢位）(c.f. fundamental position: 基本肢位)，＊20 運搬肘 (or, cubital angle：肘角)

A. Tennis elbow（lateral epicondylitis）and Thrower's elbow（medial epicondylitis）
——テニス肘（外側上顆炎）と投球肘（内側上顆炎）

Tennis elbow, as the name implies, is an injury common among tennis players, but it also affects those who carry out **respective**[*1], one-sided movements in their jobs. Problems arise in the area of the lateral epicondyle on the elbow where the muscles which extend to the fingers and wrist are attached. Pain in the lateral epicondyle when the hand is bent (**dorsiflexion**[*2]) at the wrist against resistance is a significantly important sign to justify the injury. Thrower's elbow and **golfer's elbow**[*3] are similar to tennis elbow, but much less severe. Symptoms are located at the medial epicondyle of the elbow. This injury is common among **javelin throwers**[*4] and **baseball bowlers**[*5] as well as those who turn their forearm inward vigorously when the wrist is bent. There is a severe pain when the medial epicondyle **is subject to pressure**[*6] (tenderness), and the hand is bent downward (**palmar flexion**[*7]) at the wrist against resistance.

Notes: ＊1 利き手の，＊2 背屈（付録参照），＊3 ゴルフ肘，＊4 槍投げ選手，＊5 投手，＊6 押されると（be exposed to），＊7 掌屈

B. Loose bodies in the elbow joint (osteochondritis dissecans)
——肘関節の遊離体（離断性骨軟骨炎）

This symptom is also seen in those who do throwing movements or heavy **manual labor**[*1], when the elbow is exposed to a considerable load - especially during forward movement when the arm is **relaxed and decelerating**[*2]. This can cause the convex radial head to come into violent contact with - even injure - the lateral portion of the capitulum. It may detach cartilage together with a fragment of the underlying bone from the articular surface and form a **loose body**[*3] in the joint. **Osteo-arthritis**[*4] may also follow the symptom with a loose body.

Notes: *1 腕仕事, *2 弛緩と減速（acceleration）, *3 遊離体（ねずみ）, *4 変形性関節症

1) Patient's complaints

1. I feel pain in the upper outer part of my elbow **when I make pretend throwing movements**.　投球動作をすると
2. I feel locking when I move my elbow, so **I can't complete the movement as intended**.　思うように腕が動かない
3. I feel **something small is loose** in my joint when I move my elbow.　ねずみが走るような

2) Radiographic examinations

a) AP projection　前後方向撮影

1. Sit and extend your arm flat on the table **with the palm up** (supinated position) [leaning your body toward the outside until the surface of the forearm is parallel with the cassette].　手のひらを上にして（回外位）［前腕表面がカセッテと平行になるまで体を傾けて］

b) Lateral position　側方向撮影

1. Bend your elbow to 90 degrees with **your thumb side up** [so that the oracranon process can be seen in profile] (**Fig. 13**).　親指側を上に向けて（rado-ulnar projection：橈尺方向撮影）
2. Keep the thumb side of your right hand up and place **two fingers of your left** hand under your right hand [so that your right forearm is kept horizontal].　2本の指（index and middle fingers）を右手の下に置いて

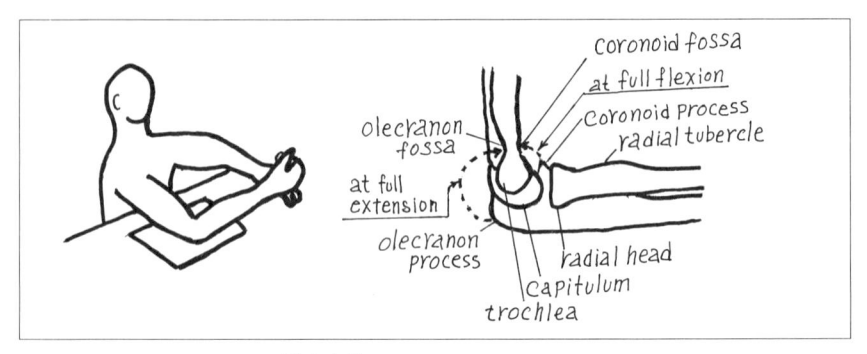

Fig. 13 Latelal position　側方向位

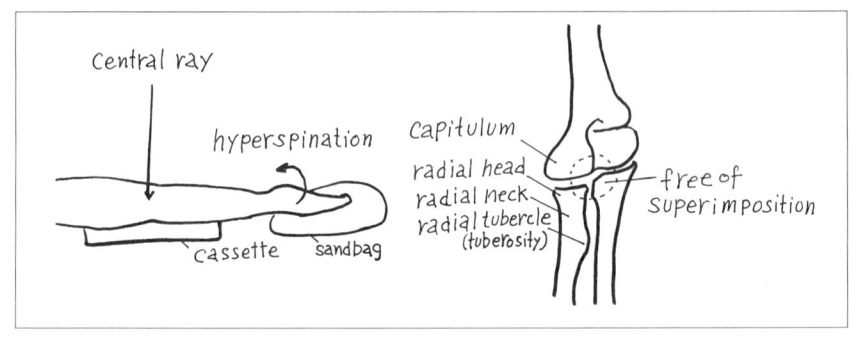

Fig. 14 Lateral obligue position　回外位

c) **Lateral oblique position**　回外位 (excessive supination：過度の回外)

This time, rotate the forearm fully outward [so that the **proximal radioulnar joint** separates with the radial head projected free of superimposition of the ulna] (**Fig. 14**). ［肘頭が尺骨と重ならずに**上橈尺関節**が開くように］

d) **Medial oblique position**　回内位 (moderate pronation)

Next, **turn** your forearm **palm down** [pronating your arm so that the anterior surface of the elbow is placed at an angle of 40 to 45 degrees with the coronoid process **projected in profile** free of superimposition] (**Fig. 15**).　掌が下を向くように［腕を回内させ，肘の表面が40〜45°になるようにして，鉤状突起が（肘頭との）重複なしに**プロファイル像として投影される**ように］

e) **Axial position**　軸位（orecranon process and distal humerus：肘頭突起と遠位上腕骨）

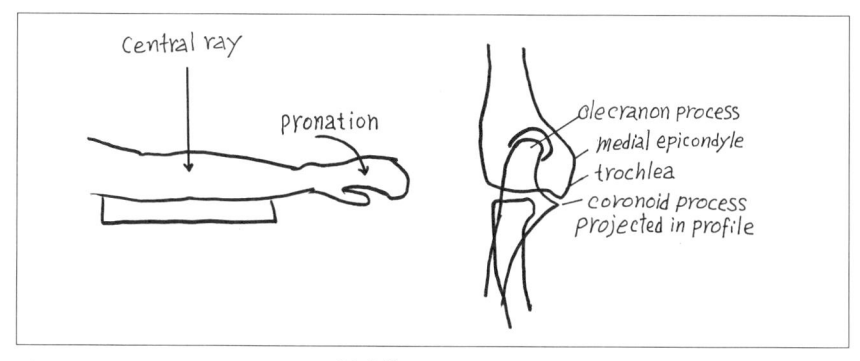

Fig. 15 medial oblique position　回内位

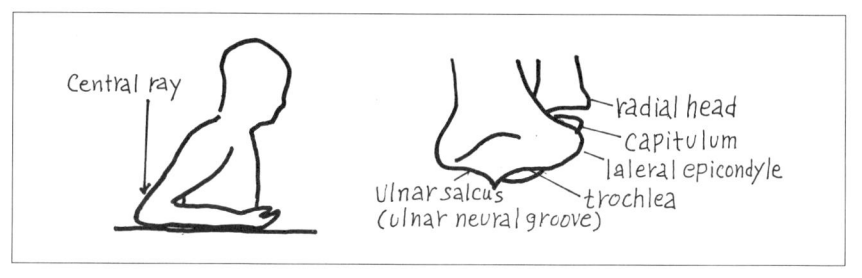

Fig. 16 Distal humerus and ulnar neural groove　遠位上腕骨と尺骨神経溝

1. Let me **direct x-rays at** the elbow head at a right angle to check if the neural tube opens wide enough [to see if the **ulnar sulcus** is not narrowed by calcification due to **radiohumeral bursitis** (tennis elbow)] (**Fig. 16**).　肘頭にX線を直角に**曝射する**（i.e. the elbow head **is exposed to x-rays** tangentially: 照射される）｜橈骨上腕骨滑液包炎が基となる石灰化によって**尺骨神経溝**の狭窄がないか（テニス肘）｜
2. **Sit sideways** with your right side against the table edge, and extend your forearm with palm up.　テーブルの端に右脇をつけて**横向きに座る**
3. Bend your arm and **lean forward a little** so the elbow **forms an angle of 45 degrees.**　肘が45°の角度になるように**少し前傾する**
4.) Rotate the palm slightly outward (supinate) to keep the upper and forearm from rotating. **Press the palm with your other hand** to keep the forearm flat on the table.　反対側の手で，その手のひらを抑えて上腕が傾かないように

3) Rehabilitation
a) **Mobility and strength exercises**　可動・ストレッチ運動

1. Place your forearm flat on the table and **press the palm of your hand against** the table top.　手のひらをテーブルに押し付ける（背掌方向）
2. Turn your forearm so that the back of your hand is pressing against the table.　手の甲をテーブルに押し付ける（掌背方向）
3. Extend your forearm until the hand **goes beyond** the table edge.　手先がテーブルの端を**超えるまで**
4. Bend your wrist down and hold it for 10 seconds.　掌屈させる（付録参照）
5. Hold a dumb-bell in your hand and simultaneously bend and straighten the elbow joint.

Quiz
A. Which bone articulates with the trochlea - the ulna or radius?
B. Which muscle fully contracts when the coronoid process tucks into the coronoid fossa, and why?
C. For a muscle to act in spination or pronation of the forearm, to which bone must it be attached, and why?
D. Who is most subject to tennis elbow, and why?
E. What makes patients feel locking when they move their elbow, and where does it come from?

Answers
A. Ulna
B. Biceps, because it spans the elbow at the anterior arm
C. Radius, because it is the radius that radiates around the ulna
D. A tennis player or those who carry out respective, one-sided movements in their jobs causing undue strain on the inner muscle of the elbow
E. A foreign body such as detached cartilage which comes from the articular surface together with a fragment of the underlying bone

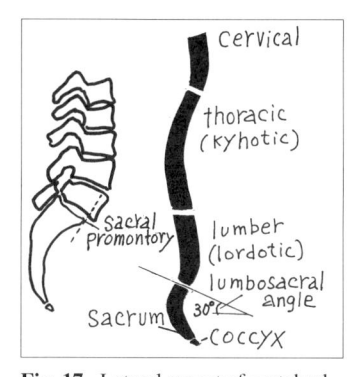

Fig. 17 Lateral aspect of vertebral column and spondylolisthesis
脊椎側面像（右）と脊椎すべり症（左）

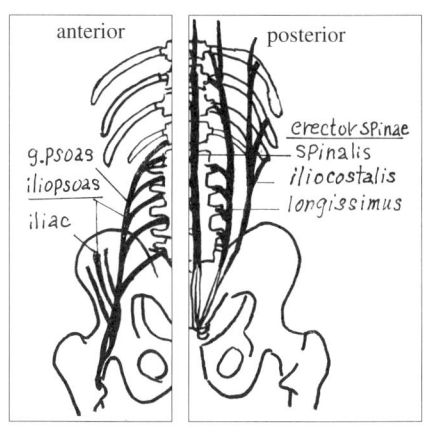

Fig. 18 Erector spinae muscles (posterior) and iliopsoas muscles (anterior aspect)
脊椎起立筋群（右肺面）と腸腰筋（右前面図）

3. Lumbar spine injuries ——腰椎損傷

Humans walk with two legs (**bipedalism**[*1]), so need vertebral curvature in order to support a heavy head and upper body with cervical and lumber spines, which are anteriorly convex, otherwise called **lordotic curves**[*2] (**Fig. 17**). On the other hand, thoracic and pelvic curves are concave interiorly (**kyphotic curves**[*3]) as compensation for keeping the posture straight. Problems often occur at the **lumbosacral junction**[*4] where the angle (lumbosacral angle) is so acute, more pronounced in females, that the lumber vertebrae slips on the sacrum beyond the **promontory** (**spondylolisthesis**[*5]). Powerful muscles include the **iliopsoas muscle**[*6] in the back which originates at the 12th thoracic vertebra and is inserted at the **lesser trochanter**[*7] and **rectus abdominis muscle**[*8], in the stomach, which is inserted at the fifth to seventh costal cartilages arising from the upper part of the pubic bone (**Fig. 18**). These muscles work together with the **gluteus maximus muscle**[*9], from the bottom, to indirectly support the lumber spine by increasing **abdominal pressure**[*10]. The rectus abdominis muscle is a powerful flexor that causes lordotic curve. Accordingly, the legs should be bent when taking x-rays so that the muscle is loose. A group of muscles called the **elector spinae muscles**[*11] contract to help extend the lumber spine with the **iliocostalis muscle**[*12] being the most effective extensor (**Fig. 19**). By doing so, the x-ray beam passes through the **intervertebral disks**[*13] as cleanly as possible.

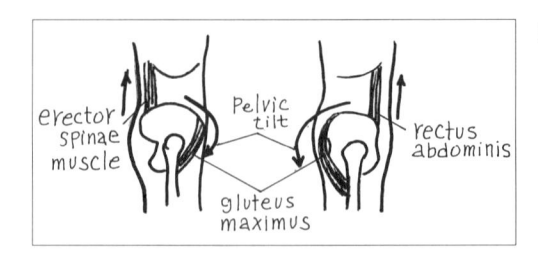

Fig. 19 Posterior (left) and anterior (right) trunk extensors and pelvic tilt　後・前体枢伸展筋と骨盤傾斜

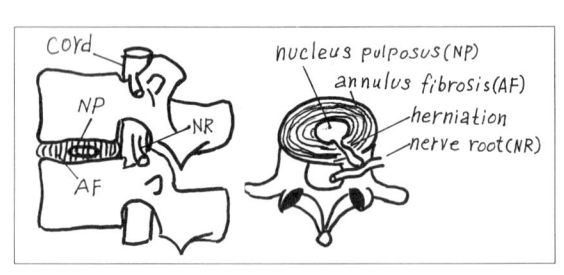

Fig. 20 Anatomic features of intervertebral discs　椎間板の解剖図

    Small elastic balls (**nucleus pulposus***14) surrounded by strong concentric sheets of fibrous tissue (**annulus fibrosis***15) in the disks make it possible for the lumber spine to move freely except during rotation, which is dependent on thoracic supine. When the annulus fiber tears as a result of trauma or **degenerative changes***16, the nucleus pulposus may **herniate***17 into a vertebral body (**slipped disks** or **herniated disks***18). This often causes back pain associated with **nerve root***19 **pain***20. However, there are many cases which cannot be determined, even though the symptoms are identical in character; these cases are called by names such as **lumbago***21, **low-back strain***22 and so on (**Fig. 20**).

Notes: ＊1 二足歩行, ＊2 前彎, ＊3 後彎, ＊4 腰仙接合部, ＊5 岬角（脊椎すべり症）, ＊6 腸腰筋〔腸骨筋（iliac muscle）と大腰筋（greater psoas muscle）からなる複合筋〕, ＊7 小転子, ＊8 直腹筋, ＊9 大臀筋, ＊10 腹圧, ＊11 脊柱起立筋, ＊12 腸肋筋（外側肋骨，横突起，腸・仙骨にV字状に着付着し，強力な外側屈筋であるが対称的に作用すると有効な伸展筋となる）, ＊13 椎間板, ＊14 髄核, ＊15 線維輪, ＊16 退行変性, ＊17 脱出する, ＊18 椎間板ヘルニア, ＊19 神経根, ＊20 （根性痛）, ＊21 腰痛症, ＊22 腰部捻挫

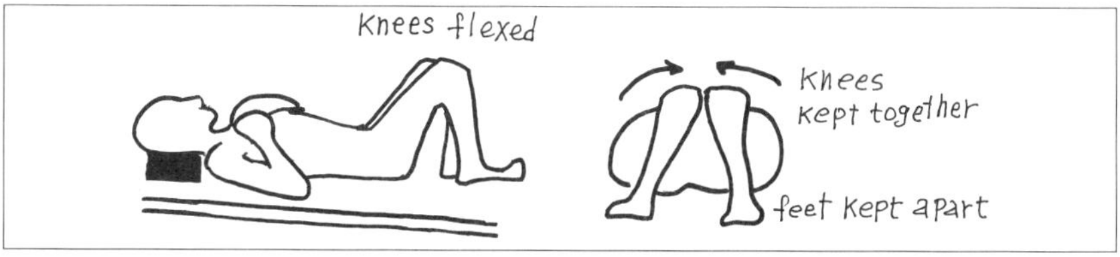

Fig. 21 Anteroposterior lumber projection　腰椎前後撮影

1) Patient's complaints

a) Cases strongly suggestive of mechanical factors　構造性背部痛が疑われる症例

① I had a sudden pain in my back when I bent over and **sneezed by chance**.　腰を曲げて**偶然にくしゃみをしたら**

② The pain is severe when I cough or **strain** my back.　背筋に**力を入れると**

③ The pain is not constant, and even disappears **at times**.　ときどき痛みが去る

④ The pain is **on and off**.　周期的に痛みがくる

⑤ The **sharp** and knife-like **pain radiates** below the knee to the ankle (**sciatic symptom**).　鋭い**痛み**が膝やくるぶしまで**放散する**（坐骨症）

⑥ I feel a sudden **stabbing pain** when I start to walk.　さしこみ

b) Other cases　神経根以外に起因する症例

① I have a **dull pain** in the buttocks.　臀部に**鈍痛**がする。

② I have constant pain at night, and can't find a **position of** comfort in bed.　夜通し痛み，寝返りをしても楽な姿勢（**安静位**）がない。

2) Radiographic examinations

a) AP projection

① Lie on your back, please.

② Bend (**flex**) your knees and **bring them up** to your chest [so your back is flat on the table] (**Fig. 21**).　屈曲／膝を立てる／［腰椎の前彎を解消するために］

@ **Psoas muscle portion** of the iliopsoas muscle **contributes to trunk flexion** only when the hip joint or femur is stabilized (like when drawing a bow to increase the **lordotic curve** of the lumber spine).　腸腰筋の**腰筋部**は股関節や大腿が安定しているときだけ**体躯の屈曲**に**貢献する**（弓を引くときのように前彎を強める）（**Fig. 18** 参照）

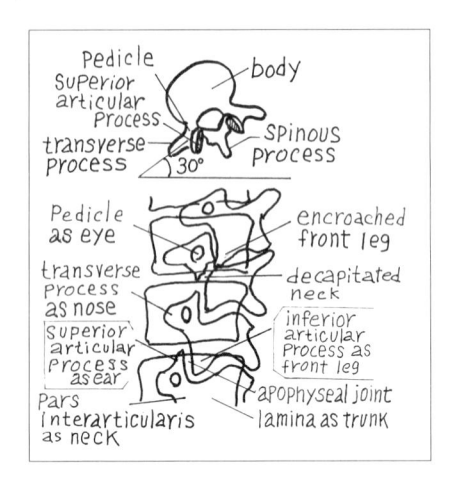

Fig. 22 Oblique position and parts of "Scotty dog". 上向き斜位と"スコッチ犬"の部分

pedicle　椎弓根
transverse/spinous process　横／棘突起
superior/ inferior articular process　上／下関節突起
apophyseal (zygapophyseal) joint　椎間関節
pars interarticularis　関節間部
lamina　椎弓板（付着部）

3 **Bring your knees together** and place your feet flat on the table.　膝を閉じる

4 Put your hands on your chest [so that they will not lie within the picture (**x-ray field**)].　［手が画面（照射野）に入らないように］

5 Take a breath, and then **let some air out** [so that the first lumber vertebra is visible with the **diaphragm** elevated].　息を吐く［横隔膜を上げて第一腰椎がみえるように］

b) **Lateral projection**

1 Turn onto your right side and **use your right arm like a pillow** [so that your vertebral column is aligned as parallel with the table as possible].　右腕を枕代わりにして［できるだけ背骨が寝台に平行になるように］

2 Bend your back and **bring** knees **up in front** [so that the vertebral column is as straight as possible].　膝を丸める［背骨ができるだけまっすぐになるように］

c) **Oblique projection（RPO: right posterior oblique）**＊　斜位方向（右後斜位）

1 Roll over onto your right side gradually (**Fig. 22**).

2 Place your arms in a comfortable position.

3 I'll adjust the angle of your back from the table at 45 degrees [for demonstration of the **articular facets** in the lumber region, and 30 degrees for the **lumbosacral facets**].　関節面／腰仙椎関節面

＊立位（upright position）では，通常この方向を左前斜位 LAO（left anterior position）と呼ぶ。

3) Radiographic findings　X線所見
a) Lateral position
1. Always check that vertebral alignment shows a smooth continuous line along the posterior edges of the vertebral bodies. Loss of lordosis is most often seen in a **prolapsed intervertebral disk** due to protective muscle spasms.　前彎の消失は防御性の筋痙攣によって生じる椎間板ヘルニアが最大の原因
2. If spondylolisthesis is suspected, attempt a second lateral view **in an upright position**.　立位で再撮影をする
3. Note deformity in all **lateral aspects of the vertebrae**.　椎体側面構造のすべての異常
4. Check also the space between vertebrae, particularly **disk space narrowing**.　椎間腔の狭小化

b) Oblique projection
1. Check that so-called "**Scotty dog shadows**" show up well to show **zygapophyseal joints**, the **transverse process** as the nose, the **superior articular process** as the ear, and the **pars interarticularis** as the neck (**Fig. 22**).　テリア像ともいう／椎間関節（or, apophyseal joint）／横突起／上関節突起／上下関節間部
2. When the patient is not oblique enough, the eye formed by the **pedicle** moves anteriorly on the vertebral body, and **vice versa** for exaggerated oblique.　逆に傾斜が大きいと犬像の目（椎弓根）は後に移動する
3. In spondylolisthesis, a forward slip of the body may **decapitate** the neck of the dog below and its front paw **encroaches on** the broken neck.　椎体部の前方へのすべりで下の犬の首を切断し，前足が折れた首に食い込む

4) Rehabilitation
a) Mobility exercises　可動運動
Hip elevation　骨盤の挙上 (gluteus maximus muscle)
1. Lie down on your back **with your heels on a chair (Fig. 23)**.　椅子の上に踵を乗せる
2. **Squeeze your buttocks** together and lift and lower your pelvis at a rapid pace.　おしりをすぼめて骨盤を速めに上下させる
3. This time, lie down on the floor with your knees bent and feet flat on the floor.
4. Place a ball between your knees and **press the knees against the ball**. Repeat the quick up-and-down motion of the pelvis again.　膝でボールを挟みつけて

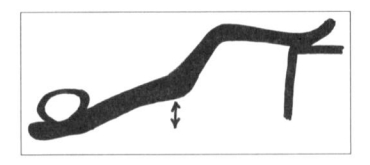

Fig. 23

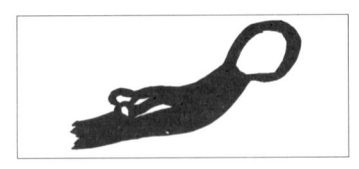

Fig. 24

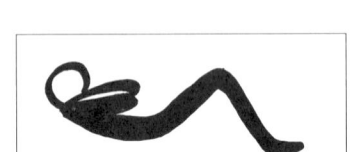

Fig. 25

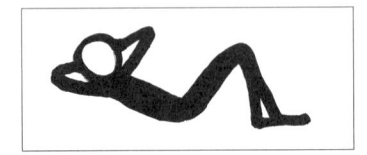

Fig. 26

b) **Strength exercises**　　筋力運動

(1)**Back extension**　　背筋の伸展 (erector spinae muscle group)

　① Lie face down **with your hands on your lower back (Fig. 24)**.　　両手を腰の後に回して

　Raise the upper part of your body so that your **chin and chest are off the floor** and hold this position for several seconds.　　顎と胸を床から浮かせるように

　② This time, **stretch out your arms in front** of you for a stronger affect.　　両手を前に突き出す

　③ Repeat the same exercise above, but extend holding time in raised position to ten seconds.

(2)**Exercise for abdominal muscles**　　腹筋（直腹筋と外方腹斜筋）の強化

　(rectus abdominis muscle and external oblique muscles)

c) **Isotonic exercise**　　等張性運動：ストレッチ

　① Lie down on your back with your knees bent and feet flat on the floor, **arms crossed over your chest** and hands on your shoulders (**Fig. 25**).　　胸の前で腕を交差させて両肩をつかむ

　② Raise your head and the upper body and hold this position for several seconds.

　③ This time, clasp your hands behind your neck (**Fig. 26**).　　両手を頭の後ろで組む

　④ Raise your head and upper body, rotate **to the right**, and hold this position for several seconds.　　左の肩を床から浮かせて，左側の上半身が**右**を向くように

　⑤ Most of your back should be in contact with the floor.

Chapter V. Musculoskeletal Injuries   131

Fig. 27   **Fig. 28**   **Fig. 29**

6 Repeat the same exercise in the opposite direction.
   @ The **external oblique** muscle bilaterally bends the trunk but unilaterally bends and rotates to the opposite side. The right side of the muscle rotates the right shoulder toward the left.　外方斜筋は両方では体躯を屈曲させるが，片側では側屈や反対側への回旋筋となる。右側の筋は右肩を左側に回すことになる

d) Static stretching exercises　ストレッチ

(1)**Abdominal curl**　体躯の巻き上げ (rectus adominis, external & internal oblique)
　1 Lie down on your back with your knees bent (**Fig. 27**).
　2 Grasp your knees with your hands and **form your body into a ball**.　両膝を抱え込んでボールのように丸くなる
　3 This time, **extend** your arms **up straight** from the floor.　床の上に両手を**伸ばす**
　4 If possible, **roll over far enough** that your toes reach the floor when your legs are stretched (**Fig. 28**).　脚のストレッチのため，両足のつま先が床につくまで**体を丸める**
　　@ The **internal oblique muscle** acts oppositely to the external oblique muscle in rotating the trunk to the same side when one side contracts; that is, the right side of the muscle rotates the right shoulder to the right.　内方斜筋は片側が収縮すると回旋筋となり，右側の筋は右肩を右側に回す

(2)**Pelvic rotation**　骨盤の回旋 (iliopsoas muscle)
　1 Lie down on your back, bend your right leg and cross **it over the left one** by turning your hips (**Fig. 29**).　右脚を曲げて**左脚の上に交差させる**
　2 Using your left hand, pull up your right leg as far as possible.
　3 Both your shoulders should be in contact with the floor.
　4 Hold the position for several seconds.　外側可動域で

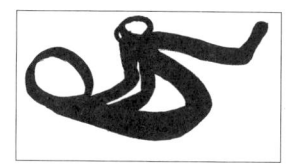

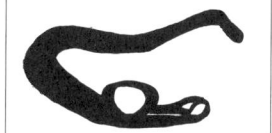

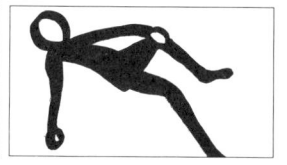

Quiz

A. Why is the lumber spine movable in all directions except rotation with the help of

respective muscles?
B. Why does the lordotic curve lessen when the knee is flexed in a supine position? (See **Figs. 17** and **19**)
C. Why does slipped disk (herniation) occur?
D. When taking x-rays of the lumbosacral joint, the central ray must travel 30 degrees off the horizontal axis (cephalad/ caudad) to pass parallel to the lumbosacral angle? (See **Fig. 17**) Select the correct direction in the parenthesis.
E. When the fifth lumber vertebra slides forward on the corresponding surface of the sacrum, what part of the sacrum becomes the reference point for the spondylolisthesis?

Answers
A. The intervertebral discs are composed of elastic balls called nucleus pulposus surrounded by strong concentric sheets of fibrous tissue (annulus fibrosis). Each vertebral body can swing on the pulposus as an axis.
B. Because the strongest trunk flexor, the rectus abdominis muscle, is loosened and the strongest back extensor, the erector spinae muscle, contracts
C. The nucleus pulposus is under constant pressure. If the annular fibers tear as a result of trauma or generative changes, the nucleus dislocates.
D. Cephalad
E. Sacral promontory　　仙骨岬角

4. Knee injuries　　——膝関節部の損傷

The various ligaments of the knee joint cooperate so that the stability of the joint is maintained. An impact against the lateral side of the knee joint which **forces the joint inward**[1] is considerably more common (90 percent of injuries) than an impact against the **medial side of the knee joint**[2] (10 percent of injuries). Knee joint injuries are subject to the degree of the impact. If the impact is **mild**[3], the deeper portion of the medial collateral ligament ruptures first, followed by superficial ruptures. A **stronger impact**[4] may rupture the anterior **cruciate ligament**[5]. An **extremely violent**[6] impact can cause posterior damage which can involve damage to the medial **meniscus**[7] and **collateral ligament**[8], as well as the anterior and posterior cruciate ligaments. The overall effect would be medial as well as **anteroposterior instability**[9] between the tibia and the femur (**Fig. 30**).

Chapter V. Musculoskeletal Injuries

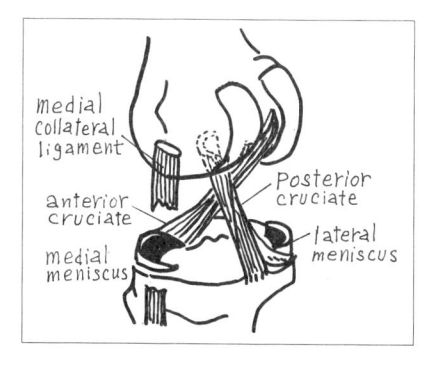

Fig. 30 Particular defense system of knee
膝の防御機構

medial collateral ligament
内側側副靭帯
anterior/ posterior cruciate
前/後十時靭帯
medial/ lateral meniscus
内側/外側半月板

On the other hand, a deep rupture of the medial collateral ligament only shows medial instability characterized by **wobbling***10 of the lower leg when the knee joint is flexed at an angle of 20 degrees. The lateral side of the knee is most often affected by an impact when the foot is bearing a load and the knee joint is slightly bent. The menisci also stabilize the joint throughout its range of motion and contribute to its limitation of motion. They also serve as shock absorbers between the femur and tibia. Note that the fibula has no articulation with the knee joint. The stress of bearing weight mainly involves the medial compartment of the knee, and it is usually in this area that primary **osteoarthritis***11 first occurs. Secondary osteoarthritis may follow ligament and meniscus injuries, **recurrent dislocation***12 of the patella, **osteochondritis dissecans***13 etc. Overweight, **degenerative changes***14 with aging and overwork are common factors in such injuries. Some knee problems are caused by a disturbance of alignment called **bow leg***15 which results from subluxation of the hip joint and creates a larger **shaft angle***16. In the case of osteoarthritis, the articular cartilage degenerates progressively, flaking off into the joint and thereby producing **space narrowing***17. Furthermore, **subarticular bone***18 becomes **eburnated***19 and often small **marginal osteophytes***20 appear in radiography.

Notes: ＊1 （外側からの）内方向圧迫（varus stress）, ＊2 外反（in valgus）, ＊3 軽度, ＊4 中程度（moderate）, ＊5 十字靭帯, ＊6 極度の（severe）, ＊7 半月版, ＊8 側副靭帯, ＊9 前後動揺, ＊10 動揺する, ＊11 変形性関節症, ＊12 習慣性脱臼, ＊13 離断性骨軟骨炎, ＊14 退行性変化, ＊15 O脚（内反膝）(genu varum), cf. X脚（外販膝）knock knee（genu valgum）, ＊16 頸体角, ＊17 関節腔の狭小化, ＊18 関節下皮質, ＊19 硬化, ＊20 辺縁骨棘

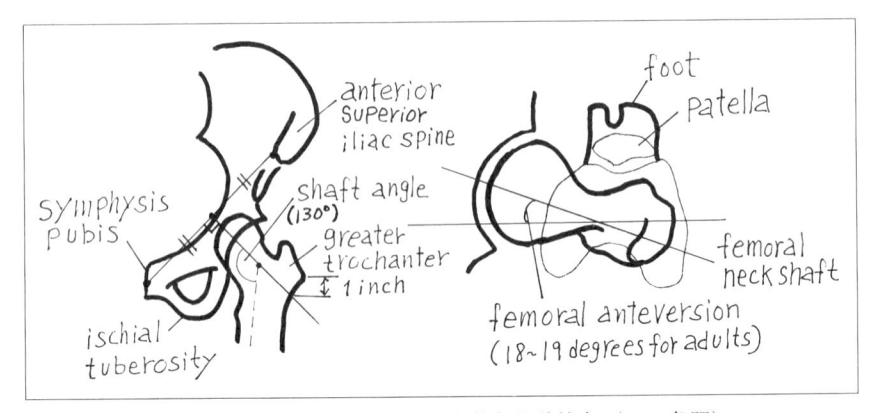

Fig. 31 Shaft angle and femoral anteversion　頸体角と前捻角（P145参照）

A. Knee joint ——膝関節
1) Radiographic examination
a) AP projection
1. Extend your leg and **rotate it inward a little** so that your **little toe is straight up** [to correct **anteversion** at the femoral neck and to ensure the kneecap faces inward] **(Fig. 31)**.　第2趾が上を向くように脚をやや内に回して［大腿頸部の**前捻角**（18〜19°）を正して膝蓋骨が内側を向くように］
2. Don't rotate the hip. The knee's rotation depends on the hip joint.
   @ The hip has a **ball-and socket joint** which permits free movement in all directions in contrast to the knee joint, a **hinge-type joint**, which only allows flexing and extending.　球関節／蝶番（ちょうつがい）関節

b) Lateral projection
1. Turn on your right side.
2. Bend your left leg **and cross it over in front** of your right leg **(Fig. 32)**.　右前に渡す
3. Let me bend the right leg enough (30 degrees), so the patella is positioned well.
   @ At this angle, **high-riding or low-riding patella** is evaluated. The more the knee is bent the higher the tension of the patellar tendon pulling the patella down on the **condyle-trochlea** (See Fig. 1).　膝蓋高位・低位／大腿顆滑車

c) Posterior anterior weight-bearing position（Rosenberg et al.）　後・前方向荷重位（ロゼンバーグ法）

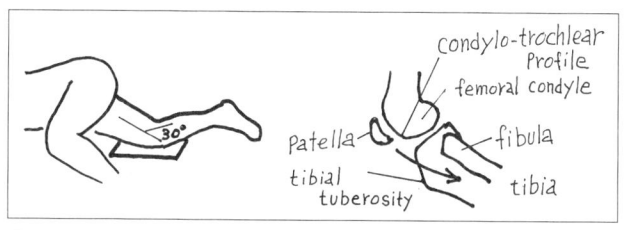

Fig. 32 Movement of patella on the femur related to knee flexion　膝屈曲による膝蓋骨の動き

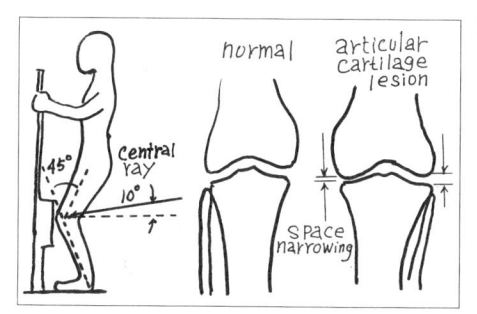

Fig. 33 Rosemberg weight-bearing position　ローゼンバーグ荷重法

1. Stand and place your feet **straight ahead**, grasp both edges of the **grid device**, and separate the feet enough for **good balance** (**Fig. 33**).　まっすぐ正面向けて／フィルム収容装置／バランスを保つため
2. Let me bend your legs at an angle of 45 degrees.
3. Stand straight and **distribute your weight equally on both feet**.　両足に等しい体重をかけて
4. Hold the position until I tilt the x-ray tube down so the central beam cleanly passes through the knee joint.

2) Rehabilitation

a) Mobility exercise　可動運動

Knee flexion　膝の屈曲　Flexors (hamstring muscle group　ハムストリング)

1. Lie down on your back on the floor with the foot of your **injured leg up against a wall** (**Fig. 34**).　怪我をした足を上げて壁に押しつけて

    Let your foot **slide downward** and at the same time bend your knee.　膝を曲げながら足をずり下げる

Fig. 34

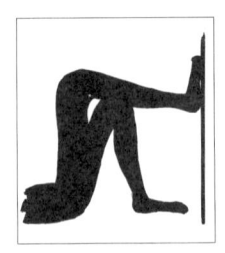

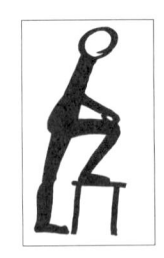

Fig. 35

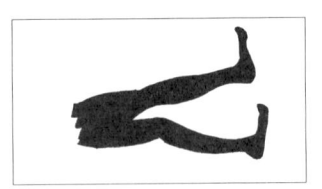

Fig. 36

2. This time, stand with the foot of your injured leg on a chair (**Fig. 35**).　今度は、立って足を椅子の上に置く

Slowly **stretch forward** so that the knee is bent. Hold the position for 10 seconds.　背筋を伸ばしたまま前傾させる

@ As the **biceps femoris** in the hamstring muscle group is **a two-joint muscle** spanning the hip and knee joint, when the knee is flexed the hip is extended.　大腿二頭筋は2関節筋だから

b) Strength exercise　筋力運動

Knee extension　膝の伸展

Extensors (quadriceps muscles：大腿四頭筋)

1. Lie down on your back, with your legs straight (**Fig. 36**).

Bend the foot of your injured leg **up**, flex your thigh muscle and **lift** your leg **with the knee straight**. Hold the position for 10 seconds.　の背屈 (dorsiflexion) ／脚を曲げてからまっすぐ伸ばして持ち上げる

2. This time, raise and lower your leg 10 times keeping the knee straight.

@ As the **rectus femoris muscle** in the quadriceps muscle group is also a two-joint muscle, when the knee is extended the hip is flexed.　大腿直筋も2関節筋だから

c) Static stretching exercise　ストレッチ

(1)**Exercise for extensors**　伸展筋の運動

1. Lie face down and grasp the ankle of your injured leg with one hand (**Fig. 37**). Attempt to straighten the leg **against the resistance of** your hand for several seconds.　手の力に逆らって

Chapter V. Musculoskeletal Injuries

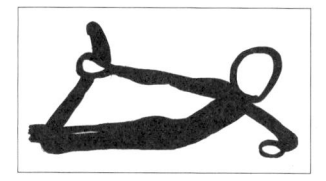

Fig. 37

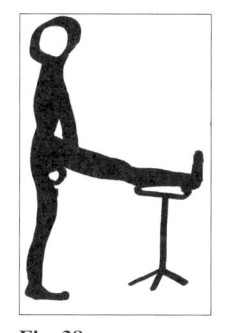

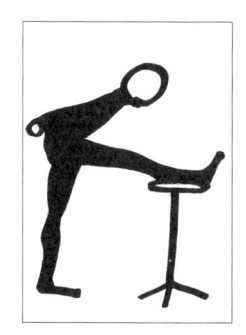

Fig. 38

Fig. 39

② This time, stretch by **pulling the foot as far up as possible** for several seconds. 足をできるだけ背屈先させたままで10秒間ストレッチをする。

③ Repeat the exercise in a standing position, **applying resistance to your leg with both hands**.　両手に脚が逆らうように

(2) **Exercise for flexors**　屈曲筋の運動

① Put your injured leg on a table (**Fig. 38**).　丸椅子の上に怪我をした方の足を置く

Straighten both legs **with the foot** of your healthy leg **pointed straight ahead** and your back kept straight.　足の低屈 (plantar flexion)

Press your heel against the surface of the table for several seconds.　かかとを押しつける

② This time, stretch for several seconds by **bending the foot** of your injured leg **up**, **while** you stretch and **bend forward from the hips** with a straight back (**Fig39**). つま先を立てて／立ったままストレッチをして，腰だけを曲げる。

For further stretching, bend the knee of your healthy leg.　このとき正常側の膝を曲げると，ストレッチの強度が増す。

B. Patella and patellofemoral joint ——膝蓋骨と膝蓋大腿関節

1) Patient's complaints

① I feel pain when walking up and down stairs, especially walking down. ＠ Compression forces between the patella and femur increases with increased knee flexion. Moreover, when descending stairs, the increased knee flexion is controlled by the quadriceps alone since one is unable to lean forward in contrast to the case when

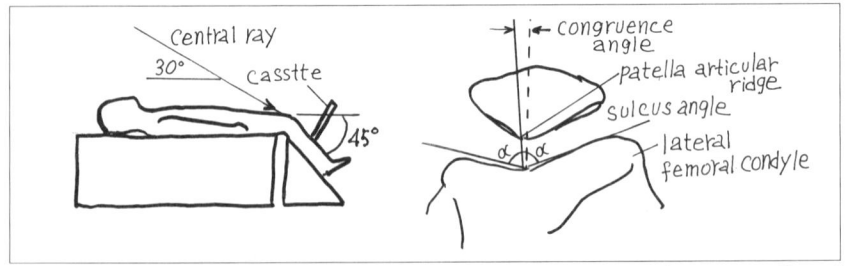

Fig. 40 Marchant method for determining congruence angle (i.e. relation between patella and intercondylar sulcus)　膝蓋大腿関節適合性を調べるためのマーチャント撮影法（膝蓋骨と顆間溝の関係）

ascending stairs.　前傾
② I find it difficult sitting with the knee bent.　正座する（cf. sit cross-legged: 胡坐をかく）
③ I feel pain when I rise from a sitting to a standing position, let alone squatting.　ましてしゃがむなんてできない

2) Radiographic examination
a) Merchant method　マーチャント法
① Lie on your back with your knees at the end of the radiographic table (**Fig. 40**).
② Lower your legs along the tilted table and let me **strap both legs together** around the calves, so that your legs do not rotate.
③ This time, your legs are bent 45 degrees. The same angle will be used for reproducibility during **follow-up examinations**.　両脚をそろえて紐で縛る／追跡検査
④ Relax your muscles around the knees (**femoral quadriceps**), or an abnormal (subluxed) patella, **if any**, may be diagnosed normal because it will be pulled back into the original position (**intercondylar sulcus**).　大腿四頭筋／もし膝蓋骨に亜脱臼があったにしても／顆間溝
⑤ Be patient, please. This method is the most complicated and takes longer than the other methods for showing the kneecap in profile (**tangential or axial view**) but most reliable for **radiographic measurements** of relationships in the area where subluxation and dislocation of the kneecap most frequently occur.　接線または軸位／画像計測

Chapter V. Musculoskeletal Injuries

@ The traditional "skyline" view of having the knee flexed at an **acute angle** doesn't visualize these relationships since instability of the patella occurs close to full extension.　鋭角 (cf. obtuse angle=鈍角)

b) **Hughston method**　　ヒューストン法

1. Lie on the table on your stomach and raise your leg, please.
2. Rest the instep (dorsal surface) of your foot on the bar (so that leg is elevated 60 degrees from the table).
3. This time, the x-ray beams (**central ray**) will pass downward (45° cephalad) aimed at the narrow space beneath the patella, so be sure not to move.　中心線

   @ This method is advocated since instability of the patella occurs close to full extension. In this case reference of the sulcus angle is 118° (Cf.138° in Marchant method in P. 142)

3) Rehabilitation
Stretching and pool exercises

1. Sit on the floor with your legs extended and push the kneecap slowly up and down, and left to right, with your thumb and fingers. Especially **pushing inward** and upward is effective.　膝蓋骨外側部を押し**内側**に押しこむ（i.e. varus stress）

   @ As fatigue and aging advances, the patella is said to tend to sag causing pressure on the outer surface of the femur. Therefore, the latero-inferior part of the **patellar tendon** hardens.　膝蓋靭帯の外底部が硬化する

2. Walk in a pool and swim with a moderate **flutter kick**.　バタ足
3. **if pain allows**, sink yourself to an underwater squatting position and stand up 痛くなければ

Quiz

A. Which bones make up the knee joint?
B. Which cruciate ligament prevents the tibia from moving anteriorly?
C. Which muscles extend the hip and flex the knee and which muscles do just the opposite?
D. Why must the leg be rotated inward when taking x-rays of AP knee?
E. What is demonstrated by Rosenberg's weight-bearing position?
F. What method is most reliable for radiographic measurement of the relationship between the patella and patellofemoral joint?

G. Which part of the knee is usually affected first by osteoarthritis?

Answers
- A. Femur and tibia
- B. Anterior cruciate ligament
- C. The hamstring muscles, the rectus femoris muscles
- D. The rotation corrects the anteversion at femoral neck
- E. Joint space narrowing due to articular cartilage disorders
- F. Merchant method
- G. The medial compartment

Relevant expressions and additional phrases

1) Expressions of definitions　　定義の表現

1. The anatomical position **is defined as** a standing position with the eyes facing forward, feet parallel and close together and hands at the sides of the body with the palms facing forward (**Fig. 41**).　　解剖学的正面（肢位）の説明
2. The fundamental position is the same as the anatomical position except that the palms face the sides of the body.　　基本肢位と解剖学的正面の違い
3. Abduction **refers to** movement of a body part away from the central axis of the body, as opposed to adduction being a movement of a body part toward the axis.　　外転と内転の説明
4. Caudal, caudad and inferior **are referred to as** parts close to the feet, as opposed to cranial, cephalic and superior being parts closer to the head.　　尾（足）方向と頭方向の説明
5. Proximal **means** toward the trunk of the body, as opposed to distal meaning away from the trunk.　　近位と遠位の説明

2) Geometric expressions　　幾何学的表現

a) Scapulohumeral rhythm　　肩甲上腕リズム

1. Scapulohumeral rhythm is an integrated motion between the shoulder girdle and shoulder joint in which the scapula rotates upward a given degree with respect to humeral elevation.
2. In a normal case, with the palpable medial margin of scapula as the **reference line** (RL), scapula tilt from the sagittal plane forms an S angle at a constant ratio of one to two compared to the SH angle (See **Fig. 2**).

Chapter V. Musculoskeletal Injuries   141

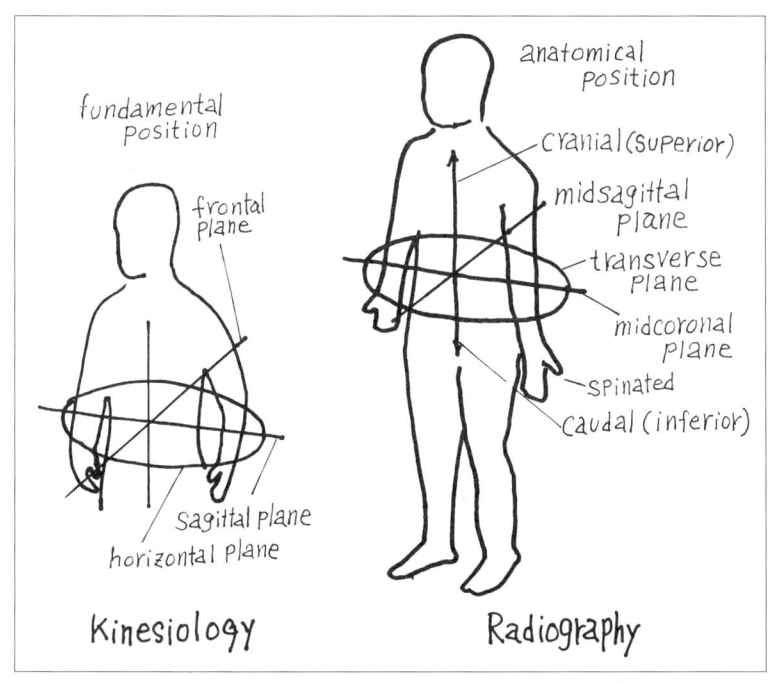

Fig. 41 Anatomical position in radiography and fundamental position in kinesiology
放射線画像学における解剖学的肢位と運動学における基本的肢位（肘90°屈曲位では機能的基本肢位と呼ぶ）

3. When the humerus is abducted 90 degrees, the S and SH angles result in 30° and 60°, respectively, with one becoming a **complementary angle** to the other. At the uppermost elevation (180° abduction) of the humerus, the angles are 60° and 120°, two angles whose measures **add up to** 180° or **supplementary angles**.

4. In this position, the clavicle is elevated 60° from the horizontal line and rotates its shaft 45° in conjunction with the rhythmic motion. When one assists in elevating a patient's humerus or applying **manipulation (reduction)**, scapulohumeral rhythm must always **be taken into consideration** since the motion of each component is so subtle and closely interrelated.　参照線／余角／和が〜となる／補角（複数形）／徒手整復／互いの動きは微妙かつ密接に関連しているので，常に肩甲上腕リズムに気を配る

b) **Localization of center of the femoral neck**　大腿骨頸部中心位置

1. Clinically draw a line between the **anterior superior iliac spine** and the upper margin of the **pubic symphysis** (See **Fig. 31**).

② Draw a second line from a point one inch inferior to the **greater trochanter** to the midpoint of the previous marked line.

③ The femoral head will lie in the same plane as this line parallel to the neck with its center point in the middle. 　上前腸骨棘／恥骨結合／大転子

c) **Congruence angle** 　コングルエンスアングル（膝蓋大腿関節整合角）

① Draw two lines on an x-ray picture, taken by the Merchant method, from the highest points on the lateral and medial **femoral condyles** toward the lowest point in the **intercondylar sulcus** (See **Fig. 34**). 　大腿骨内外顆／大腿顆間溝

② These two lines form the **sulcus angle** that is around 138 degrees with a higher value being indicative of **dysplasia of lateral condyle of the femur**. 　サルカスアングル（大腿内外顆関節面角：**Fig. 34** の 2α）／大腿骨外顆の形成不全

③ Draw a line **bisecting** the sulcus angle and a second line projected from the apex of the sulcus angle through the lowest point on the apex of the **articular ridge** of the patella. 　二等分する／関節面突起稜

④ When the second line is medial to the first line or zero line, it is defined negative, and **otherwise positive**. 　最初の線（基準線）の外側だったら正とする

⑤ The normal congruence angle is **somewhat negative** and recurrent dislocation of the knee occurs at an angle of 23 degrees. 　幾分負角である

d) **Measurement of Q-angle** 　Q角の計測

① Clinically draw a line from the **tibial tuberosity** to the center of the patella (See **Fig. 12**). 　脛骨粗面

② Draw a second line **along the direction of** the quadriceps mechanism. 　～の方向に沿って

③ The angle formed by the **intersecting** of these lines represents the Q-angle. 　交わり（i.e. an included angle: 挟角）

④ The normal Q-angle is 14 degrees, with 20 degrees considered abnormal, being associated with **patellar instability** and generative changes. 　膝蓋骨不安定性

Exercises V

V-1. Answer the following question in English, using the key words below.

Why should medical staff acquire multidisciplinary knowledge in their area of expertise? 　なぜ医療スタッフは学際的な知識を身につけなければならないか。

1) not familiar with, 2) on the other hand, 3) specialist for, 4) not in a position to, 5) technical interruption, 6) multidisciplinary knowledge, 7) team medicine, 8)

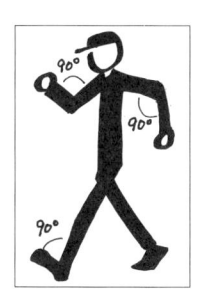

Fig. 42 How to walk for aerobic exercise
有酸素運動の歩行法

close contact with each other

V-2. Translate the Japanese into English referring to Fig. 42.
　ウォーキングの基本は，歩幅を広くとり，前に出す足首は90度に曲げて踵から着地する。後ろの足は膝を伸ばしてつま先で地面を強く蹴り，ほぼ一直線のライン上をできるだけ速く歩く。姿勢は，胸を張り背筋を伸ばし，顎を引いて頭をまっすぐにし，視線は高い位置から少し遠くを見下ろす。肘は90度に曲げ，前後に大きく振る **(Fig. 42)**。

V-3. Translate the English into Japanese taking the parts in bold letters into consideration.
　As advanced and complicated as medicine is, it demands that medical doctors and related professionals from various specialties function as teams centered on individual patient needs. Commonly known as "team medicine," staff members must possess multidisciplinary knowledge and skills in ensuring smooth and effective patient care. The team approach greatly assists members in sharing critical information and achieving closer cooperation. **The last thing they should do is** forget the fact that a patient is a member of the team medicine approach. Without his/ her cooperation or a positive will to participate, any effort by the other team members **might be to no avail**.

Example answerは巻末（付録の前）に掲載

Chapter VI.

Debate and discussion
ディベートと会議

1. Debate ——ディベート

Proposition 1: Medical stuff (MS) should have a fixed assignment position
論題1：医療スタッフの職場は固定されるべきである

Two teams, the **affirmative side***1 (**pro**) represented by Mr. A and the **opposing side***2 (**con**) represented by Mr. B, are participating in a debate. The **proposition***3 is that medical staff (MS) should have **fixed assignment positions***4. **Medical staff***5 refers to staff who are working in a **specific medical-related field***6 such as RN, RT, PT, OT, MT, CET, ST and so forth. Therefore, the definition of a fixed assignment position differs greatly according to the particular field. Taking radiological technology for example, it encompasses the three following separate and distinct **departments***7: radiography, radiotherapy and nuclear medicine. And even in each department many **workplaces***8 exist. For radiography, for example, you have CT, MRI, US, GI, angiography and others. Rotation of assignment, in such a case, would most likely mean an **intradepartmental***9 rotation. **Interdepartmental***10 rotation, on the other hand, may mean moving between different departments, from floor to floor, as the case with a nurse. For an MT, each laboratory is independent with no rotation except for special cases. The following situation involves an RT rotation, but one should keep in mind that other cases could apply.

Notes: *1 肯定側, *2 反対側, *3 論題, *4 固定職場, *5 医療従事者 (co-medical or allied medical), *6 以下の各職種：RN (registered nurse：看護師)・RT (radiologic(al) technologist：診療放射線技師)・PT (physical therapist：理学療法

士)・OT(occupational therapist:作業療法士)・MT(medical technologist:臨床検査技師)・CET(clinical engineering technician:臨床工学技士)・ST(speech therapist:言語療法士)・その他,＊7 放射線診断・放射線治療・核医学検査室,＊8 以下の各部署:CT・MRI・超音波・消化管検査・血管造影・その他,＊9 部署内交代勤務,＊10 部署間交代勤務

Moderator　司会者

We would like to debate the **resolution** that medical staff should have a fixed assignment position. For a long time, there has been discussion on this topic here and there around the world, but a definitive decision has not yet been made. In most cases, the decision has **rested upon** the circumstances in which a staff member is working. The important point in our debate today is not that we draw a conclusion but that we **bring out** by a process of **inquiry and advocacy**, issues we can pinpoint. Each of the debaters has chosen the side that they wish to defend. They must prove each point in order to convince the audience.　"医療従事者の職場は固定すべきである"と**決められた**論題／環境**次第**である／何が争点の中核であるかを**討議・論争**を通して**明確**にする

Before we begin, I would like to first **go over** the rules. The **time structure** is a five-minute **constructive speech**, a three-minute **cross-examination**, and a final five-minute **rebuttal**. In the opening speech, the affirmative side should include all important points, plans, and advantages. During its presentation, the opposing team cannot interrupt by asking questions or making objections. All responses must wait until the cross-examination starts.　ルールを**確認する**／時間構成／基調演説／反対尋問／反駁

Then comes the cross-examination of the affirmative by the opposing side. The purpose of the cross-examination is to clarify arguments and focus on important remarks from the opposing side that the **examiner** can use as **attack objectives** in the rebuttal that will come next. The opposing side then states its case in its opening constructive speech. Its task, however, is to present **rational arguments** opposing the resolution. It does this by focusing on the weakness of the proposition itself, rather than on the affirmative side's opening statements. The rebuttal comes later.　**質問者**は相手側の重要な発言に的を絞り,それを後続の反駁で**攻撃材料**にする／**論理的な議論**(相手側の主張に反対するより,論題の持つ弱点を突く)

Chapter VI. Debate and Discussion 147

The affirmative side, in turn, is then given the opportunity to cross-examine the opposing side. You are reminded that in this debate **silence is NOT golden**, but is considered to be a sign of acceptance. What you shouldn't forget is that the examiner cannot attack the debater's personality or attack him / her emotionally. After the cross-examination by the affirmative side comes the **opposing rebuttal**, during which the opposing side attacks the affirmative side's arguments and emphasizes the **veracity** of its own arguments.

The affirmative side then has its chance to rebut in an attempt to reconstruct its case and rebuild each point of contention. Following the affirmative side's closing statement, the debate is then decided based on the merits of both side's performance.　　沈黙は金でなく承諾とみなされる／反対側の反駁／正当性を強調する

Mr. A, you may proceed.

Constructive speech of the affirmative side　　肯定側の基調演説

Mr. A: On the basis of extensive research and investigation we, of the affirmative side, completely agree with the proposition that medical staff (MS) should have a fixed assignment position. We firmly believe this **plan** is supported by several **solid arguments**, which we will now present.

First, an MS should develop strong expertise in one area by being given the opportunity to specialize in it. **With the advent of** many sophisticated machines, or machine-related technology, an MS can **keep up with** the rapid progress of this complex technology only when he/she is specialized in a given area. One may **manage** to handle high-tech machines without specializing, but the result will most likely be much less than what could be done by a specialist.　　論題／確固たる論拠／～の出現により／ついていく／何とか～できる

Second, to truly earn the title of "professional," in which an MS **has skills which are not generally held by others**, a fixed assignment is mandatory. In general, sectors of MS have not yet become fully recognized by **the public at large**. Most medical procedures have not been left to an MS **irrespective of** the simplicity. Why does a **referring doctor** have to perform tasks for an MS even though the doctor is preoccupied by his own **immediate work?** An MS won't be entrusted with responsibility as long as careless and potentially fatal errors are made and sometimes receive widespread negative publicity. If an

MS is working as a specialist in a given area, such a fundamental error won't occur. What do you mean by a specialized profession? Remember again that it is **a particular job that cannot be easily substituted by another job**. You shouldn't **base things on your own convenience**. In order to raise our **status quo**, we must make an effort to have our job clearly recognized by society.
他人には真似ることのできない技術を身につけるには／一般大衆／〜に無関係に／参照医／直の仕事で手が空かない／徐人をもって代えがたしという職業／自身の都合で物事を考える／社会的地位

Cross-examination by the opposing side　　反対側の反対尋問

Mr. B:　Your **reasoning** on the proposition is that an MS cannot become a **research-oriented staff** unless he has a fixed assignment, is that correct?　　推論／研究中心の

Mr. A:　Not always. Generally, I mean.

Mr. B:　**Wishy-washy** answer. OK, do you think such an MS as you said is always preferable as an MS?　　煮えきらない

Mr. A:　That depends. Mr. B, you are asking questions for which there are **no clear-cut answers**.　　白黒いずれかを極端に求めている

Mr. B:　Well, don't you think your idea is rather simplistic? How does an MS decide his or her area to specialize in from the beginning?

Mr. A:　They don't decide from the beginning. They decide after a couple of years in which they rotate through several different areas.

Mr. B:　Would you explain what you mean when you said that an MS would **fall behind** the rapid progress of new technology if the proposition was denied? Isn't it **true, instead**, that he or she would **fail to** keep up because he or she is not being exposed to other MS members and experiences?　　遅れをとる／反対ではないか／〜できない

Mr. A:　I mean an MS who works his or her assignment **in depth**, not just **superficially here and there**.　　深く〜する／浅く広くでなく

Mr. B:　Do you think that a narrowly-specialized MS is welcomed by an employer?

Mr. A:　Certainly. With the **proliferation of sophisticated machines**, employers will want more specialists.　　高度機器の普及につれて

Constructive speech of the opposing side　反対側の基調演説

Mr. B: The opposing position in this debate will be two-fold: first, the plan is unbelievable; and second, it is **irrelevant in relation to Japanese society**.

Let's talk about the first issue. The affirmative side makes its first argument that an MS cannot develop strong expertise unless that person is specialized in a particular area. The opposing position here is that an MS will become more motivated to absorb knowledge by rotating and being exposed to more advanced technology that has a significant impact on our profession.　日本の社会になじまない

The second argument the affirmative side makes is that we don't **deserve being called professionals** unless the proposition is approved. First of all, I find this extremely hard to swallow. Our view of what is going on in a narrow field is that the more an MS specialized in that narrow field, the more he/she seems to neglect the profession as a whole. **This calls to mind a simple truism**-that a narrow field too often **signals** a narrow mind.　プロフェッショナルと呼ばれるに値しない／よく言われているように／動機となる

The opposing side would like to state as its third and last argument that the plan does **not apply well to the Japanese social fabric**. We as a people are still accustomed to working at one location for our entire professional lives. What if a vacancy occurs in a department? Can it be easily filled by a specialist from another hospital? A trans-hospital move is not as easily done here as in the U.S., where such moves are far more **commonplace**.　日本の社会構造にマッチしない／当たり前

Cross-examination by affirmative side　肯定側の反対尋問

Mr. A: We notice you tend to expand the proposition **as you see fit**. This debate is **over the feasibility** of confining an MS to a specific area within one of the several departments.　自分勝手に／可能性について

Mr. B: What we are saying to you is that you can't narrowly define a job. Let's take the **radiation therapy department** as an example. How can you restrict someone to an area as narrow as **external beam therapy** or **brachytherapy**? 放射線治療部／外部照射／密封小線源治療

Mr. A: But you can. In the U.S., they have brachytherapy specialists.

Mr. B: This isn't the U.S.

Mr. A: You attempted to refute before that the specialization weakens the union of MS members. Isn't it different from being highly-recognized by the general public?

Mr. B: We have never intended to unite ourselves as the **former JR labor union** did, in the past, and failed to get support from the citizens. Of course, we agree that individual effort is highly important. However, a well-organized and **coherent society** of an MS group is the most efficient way to realize our expectations.　以前の国鉄労組／団結した組織

Mr. A: To us it is the individual effort of dedicated people that is the most important **stepping stone** to heightened professionalism and public appreciation of the important job we do.　地位の向上への重要な足がかり（一里塚）

Me. B: You are too idealistic. Like it or not, an active organization is an unavoidable necessity.

Rebuttal speech of affirmative side　肯定側の反駁

Mr. A: We of the affirmative position feel that the objections of the opposition are just not well thought out.

First, they argue that rotating between different fields motivates an MS to absorb new knowledge. We have several arguments against this opinion.

Our first example is this: let's consider a clinical practitioner who **hangs out a shingle** which identifies him as a surgeon as well as a physician. Next door, another surgeon identifies himself as a **head and neck specialist**. So which would you visit if you came down with a thyroid condition? Which do you think takes a more serious approach toward disease?　外科と内科の看板を掲げる／頭頸単科

The second example is of some medical professionals who are hired as specialists from the beginning. Each specialist has a certain expertise and has recently been highly appreciated by other medical staff and society.

The next argument of the affirmative side is that a hospital will have difficulty recruiting for a specific area. Well, apparently you have not fully understood the changes that the MS have had in their work attitudes. An increasing number of professionals no longer feel a need to remain at the same hospital. They're becoming more mobile, which is making it easier to fill hospital vacancies.

So we don't think that these arguments of the opposition are persuasive, and we remain convinced that an MS should have a fixed assignment position.

Rebuttal speech of the opposing side   反対側の反駁

Mr. B: The opposing side's basic position still is that an MS should gain wide knowledge in different fields. The affirmative side believes that Japanese workers of today tend not to stick to one company until retirement. This is contrary to our own observations. We think they still have difficulty in finding a company that has totally adopted the **merit system**, but not the **seniority promotion** and **lifetime employment systems**.　　成果主義／年功序列／終身雇用

Here we have heard the affirmative side weakly argue that we should expand the definition of the fixed position. However, the fact is that there are multiple departments already in each profession. This number is enough for the typical MS to find his or her own **niche** in which he or she can contribute the most professionally. What we have seen is that the more "specialists" we have, the more the profession is damaged, not helped. Furthermore, for a department to keep all its specialists trained at a high level of technical expertise requires a **liberal budget and the flexibility** to regularly send them to academic meetings. Remember the fact that there are about 20 specialty fields in the United States for an MS and the number is still expanding.　　適所／予算や人員の余裕が

The affirmative side argues as if a research-oriented MS can perform a routine more correctly or clinical practice more preferably than others. However, statistics concerning medical students reveal that students with high levels of **maturity**, **nonacademic achievement**, and **rapport** are two to three times more likely to receive "A" internship grades than those without these higher levels. Therefore, we believe that personal characteristics should first be taken into consideration for new medical staff members. So overall, the disadvantages of adopting the plan **outweigh** the advantages that the affirmative side claims.　　人間性，非学問的業績，信頼性に優れた医学生／〜をはるかに上回る

Moderator: Let's call the debate at this point. Now, who do you think is the winner? Ladies and gentlemen, would all those in favor of the affirmative side please raise your hands? Now, those in favor of the opposing side... Thank you. The proposition was supported (rejected) **by an overwhelming majority (marginally-decisive difference)**.　圧倒的多数で（かろうじて）

Quiz
- **A.** What are the two main issues of this debate?
- **B.** What does the affirmative side claim on each issue?
- **C.** What is the analogy used in the rebuttal of the affirmative side?
- **D.** How does the opposing side refute the affirmative side's claims?
- **E.** What is the third or last argument made by the opposing side in its constructive speech?
- **F.** Which side do you support, why?

Answers
- **A.** Developing expertise and raising status quo
- **B.** ① One must acquire knowledge or technique in depth, but not superficially.
  ② An MS should make an effort toward being highly recognized within a fixed assignment.
- **C.** Two types of surgeons
- **D.** ① An MS will become more motivated toward absorbing knowledge by rotation.
  ② The more an MS specializes in one narrow field, the more he or she fails to view the profession as a whole.
- **E.** The proposition is irrelevant to Japanese society.
- **F.** Answer either way according to your own belief.

Proposition 2: Competitive market system should be introduced to hospital administration.

論題2．病院管理に競争原理を導入すべきである

Constructive speech of the affirmative side　　肯定側の基調演説

Mr. A:　We are firmly convinced that adoption of the resolution is urgent and inevitable. By introducing the **principle of market competition** in medical care, with excellent medical institutions favored by patients and inferior ones **driven out of the market**, the quality of a nation's medical services will be enhanced.　　競争原理／優れた医療が患者に選択され，劣ったところが**淘汰される**

Chapter VI. Debate and Discussion   153

One problem with the health insurance system that has been pointed out is the **piecework system** of its operation. The more medicine is prescribed or the more medical tests are conducted, the higher the medical payments to medical institutes or practitioners become. As well as being a waste of money, over-prescription of medicine and too many medical checkups may also end up harming patients. It is wrong to think just because a hospital is run like a **joint-stock company**, it is merely pursuing profit **at the expense of** the quality of care it gives to patients. It is unreasonable to exclude the medical-care sector alone from **regulatory reforms** when all of economic and social systems are **now under review**.　出来高払い／株式会社／～の犠牲の上で／構造改革／見直しを迫られるなかで

If a competitive system is introduced, like it or not, a so-called **skill mix** will start among doctors and other medical staff in order to reduce personnel expenses. The insurance program urges hospitals to substituted a share of the doctor's work with a less expensive MS (**physician's extender**). In such a case a **nurse practitioner** would serve as a **gate keeper** for a clinic physician, and **RPA** (radiology practitioner assistant) would do **triage** or select massive films which are unnecessary for a radiologist to read. This kind of drastic cost reduction could be achieved only when each sector of professionals abandon their **vested interests** realizing " **Need knows no laws.**"　（異分野の）技術補完／医師補完者／臨床看護師／被保険患者の第一次診療者／放射線科医補完技師（super-technologist）／選別作業をする（RADS：radiographer abnormality detection system in UK）／既得権／背に腹は代えられぬ

Cross-examination by the opposing side　反対側の反対尋問

Mr. B:　Your reasoning on the proposition is that superior medical institutions will be **preferred** by patients and inferior ones **driven out of business**, by introducing the principle of market competition, is that correct?　患者に**選別され**，劣った病院はつぶれてしまう

Mr. A:　Yes, of course.

Mr. B:　If that's true, won't hospitals, in their efforts to be more competitive, risk **paring down** quality assurance programs and other quality services; and even possibly **resort to "Down coding"** and other **shady** practices?　品質保証などの質を**ないがしろにする**／"過小支払いプログラム"（過去にHMO傘下の

企業が摘発された，コンピュータに恣意的に少なめの支払額を計算させるプログラム）などの**不正手段にやむを得ず頼る**ようになる

Mr. A: It used to be, yes. But today, unfair demand for payment or unreasonable reimbursement is strictly regulated by the **CPP** (Corporate Compliance Program) system. Furthermore, a computer network system or **IHE** (Integrating the Healthcare Enterprise) is being introduced so that money-related problems become more transparent, in a sense, by automatically linking related data among concerned enterprises in addition to clinical data (see chapter 7). As you know, we have a non-profit organization **JCAH** (the Joint Commission on Accreditation of Hospitals) that is responsible for the supervision of standards of practice for hospitals. A non-accredited hospital would be avoided by knowledgeable patients. 　　（強いて訳せば）企業順守綱領／医療企業間情報統合化（7章参照）／病院資格認定合同委員会

Mr. B: Do you think that all citizens should be covered by **universal health insurance**? Is it possible in a competitive market system?
国民皆保険

Mr. A: Citizens should **cover** themselves with their own insurance because universal health insurance premiums will be reduced. In the US, **the American government has left** its own insurance systems, **Medicare** and **Medicaid**, in the hands of HMOs.　　米国政府は，連邦保健制度であるメディケア（老人医療保険）やメディカイド（貧困者医療扶助）の運営を民間保険医療組合傘下の企業に任せた。

Constructive speech of the opposing side　　反対側の基調演説

Mr. B: We urge rejection of the resolution. We think the pursuit of profit does **not fit with** the medical-care field. In the medical sector all people must be treated equally, not according to how much one can afford to pay. The government-controlled health insurance system is certainly on the verge of bankruptcy. The increase in medical fees will lessen the opportunity of adopting a system under which fees are determined, in principle, by type of sickness (**DRG**: diagnostic related group). Let's look at a case in the United States that proves how the quality of medicine is **compromised** in the name of cost reductions. So far, we haven't seen any reports that privatized hospitals are superior to nonprofit institutions. In fact, we have seen the reverse, the development of the notorious **managed health care** companies controlled by the **HMO** (Health Maintenance Organization).　なじまない／疾病群別定額払い制度（いわゆる"まるめ"）／劣化する／管理保健医療／民間保健医療組合

An HMO allocates an annual budget to each hospital or clinic according to the number of patients who pay a **premium**. This is called **capitation** by which medical service automatically restricts, or provides an incentive for patients not to visit the hospital; the less patients visit or receive service, the more profit medical providers earn. If a hospital asks for a higher-tech procedure for a patient, the company tends to urge less expensive alternatives even though the higher-tech procedure may be deemed necessary. Physicians are kept completely under the control of a company, losing **professional autonomy**.　保険料／人頭払い／専門職の自立性

I will give examples of patients complaining about this system. One patient, who was not allowed to stay longer during rehabilitation after knee surgery, reluctantly went home and **fell down the stairs**. He had to return to the hospital again. Some elderly persons, under the Medicare program, have been refused reimbursement for **medicine that used to be classified as prescription medicine**; and, as a result, have had to join bus tours to Canada in order to procure the same medicine there. This kind of inconvenience for patients is reported by the mass-media almost on a monthly basis as a special report. On the other hand, company managing directors and/or board members are paid **exorbitant salaries**.　階段から転げ落ちた／以前は処方薬として認められた薬が保険適用から外されたので／法外な報酬

Cross-examination by the affirmative side　肯定側の反対尋問

Mr. A:　Do you think you can avoid bankruptcy of the current insurance system?

Mr. B:　Listen carefully, Mr. A. I said keep the current system, but modified with a DRG payment system. A physician would have to stop ordering expensive tests if a less costly test is just **as effective**.　安価な検査で同じような効果が上がるならば

Mr. A:　It's an **easygoing way of thinking**. It's next to impossible to reduce medical expenses without any drastic change. Even if DRG were adopted, most hospitals would still **have an appetite for** expensive, high-tech equipment. Even small hospitals feel the pressure to purchase expensive technology, because owning this equipment **prevents** them **from having to** refer patients elsewhere. Moreover, a hospital that doesn't have CT or MRI units will **most likely find it difficult** to attract **top-notch** medical staff. It's a **complicated circle**. Because health care workers and patients prefer hospitals with advanced equipment, so hospitals struggle to obtain the latest technology. Certainly, DRG will help hospitals reduce anxiety to **recover their initial** cost using the equipment whether or not it is necessary simply so they can be reimbursed by the insurance system. It is no wonder about 60 percent of hospitals **operate in the red** now. Don't you think that if DRG is adopted in the current system, maybe 100 % of hospitals will fall in the red? Hospitals can't help but **resort to downsizing** their scale and/or depend on **outsourcing** for human resources, which **after all ends up** being part of the competitive market system. 　安易な考え／渇望する／よそに患者を紹介せずにすむ／まず無理であろう／腕利きの／絡み合った関係／購入費を取り戻す／赤字経営である／やむを得ず規模縮小をする／外部委託／結局〜となる

Reference　　参考
Debate terminology　　ディベート用語

1. Argument: Proving a decided claim, using reasoning, or evidence which is constructed by claim, warrant and data.　　論拠：根拠や主張を推論や証拠で証明すること。主張，論拠，データで構成される
2. Case: Negative case or affirmative case constructed by both sides.　　論旨：双方の側で組み立てられる否定論，あるいは肯定論
3. Claim: One of the three structures of arguments; synonymous with contention. 主張：三つの議論を構成する要素のひとつで，contentionと同義語
4. Constructive speech: Speech stating the main issues by both sides.　　基調演説：双方がそれぞれの主要点を述べる演説
5. Cross-examination: Questioning held after each constructive speech for the purpose of investigating the other's weak points.　　反対尋問：各々の基調演説後に行われる，相手側の弱点を見出すための質疑
6. Issue: Argument which decides whether or not the proposition is to be adopted or rejected.　　争点：論題の是非を決定する論争点
7. Need: Necessity for improving the present status quo.　　必要性：現状を改革するための必要性

⑧ Proposition: Synonymous with claim or contention in a broad sense; used as the subject of an argument in a narrow sense.　論題：広義では，claim や contention と同義語。狭義では論題を指す
⑨ Reasoning: Rationale of the warrant used to relate data to the claim.　推論：data と claim を結ぶ論拠の理由付
⑩ Rebuttal: Defense against attack in a narrow sense; in a broad sense attack and defense.　反駁：狭義では攻撃に対する防御。広義では攻撃と防御を指す
⑪ Refutation: Attack, as opposed to rebuttal which has a defense connotation.　反論：rebuttal が防御の概念を持つのに反し，攻撃を意味する

Quiz

A. How does the affirmative side claim the quality of medical services will be enhanced when market competition occurs?

B. How does the affirmative side point out the disadvantage of a piecework system for health insurance operation?

C. Why does the affirmative side claim the medical care sector alone cannot be exempted from regulatory reforms?

D. How does the affirmative side claim drastic reduction of personnel expenses will be achieved if a competitive system is introduced?

E. How does the opposing side claim the swelling of medical fees will be reduced?

F. Why does the opposing side claim physicians lose when controlled by an HMO?

Answers

A. Excellent medical institutions will be favored by patients and inferior ones will be driven out of the market.

B. The system is a cause of over-prescription of medicines and too many medical checkups that may end up harming patients.

C. Because all economic and social systems are now under review of reforms.

D. A so-called skill mix would exist in which a less expensive MS would substitute a part of medical doctor tasks.

E. By adopting a system under which medical fees are determined by the type of sickness or DRG.

F. They lose their professional autonomy.

2. Brainstorming　　　　　——ブレーンストーミング

The issue : How to avoid careless error
議題：いかにして人的エラーを減らすか

Moderator　　司会者

Human error in our hospital has become **too common to overlook** these days. It's bad, but happily it has involved only minor cases so far. That's why we have gathered here today, asking a representative to attend from each department. Let's do brainstorming to try to come up with possible countermeasures to reduce careless errors. Before starting brainstorming, I'll go over the principle rule. They say **two heads are better than one**. This is true in free discussion where one idea will lead to another person thinking up an idea, producing a synergistic effect or even **a chain reaction**, where one person's idea leads to another person's idea and a third person's idea. Maybe the third person's idea is the very important idea that you are looking for. This couldn't happen in another type of situation such as open debate or just one person thinking on his own. Again a very important factor is that all members must be treated equally so that a hierarchy doesn't exist. Such a **hierarchy** makes people say everything is going fine and that no problem exists. This type of attitude is not going to help bring about any improvements through ideas.　　見逃せない（i.e. too much to tolerate：目に余る）／三人寄れば文殊の知恵／連鎖反応／身分の上下

Moderator: Let's hear first from Mr. A because he is the **one that brought the topic up**.
　　　　　　言い出しっぺ

Mr. A:　　Nowadays, especially with the rise in medical malpractice, **lawsuits related to malpractice** are becoming more common in Japan, 767 cases were filed in 2000, **soaring to more than double the number ten years ago**. I think our hospital needs to quickly set up some type of regulation in advance before medical malpractice occurs.　　医療過誤に伴う訴訟／2000年に767件の提訴があり，**過去10年間に倍増した**

Mr. B:　　We already have a quality assurance taskforce. A quality assurance (QA) program is based on the concept that basically humans are by nature good. Will

Chapter VI. Debate and Discussion 159

you tell me how it differs from a **risk management program** in a QA program?　危機管理

Mr. A: A QA program stands on the concept that **humans are by nature good**. Even though one makes errors, he/ she can make them **a lesson for** the future. However, concerning risk management in a hospital setting, safety standards or regulations must be set up based on a more serious belief that **humans are by nature bad**, that one will never be free from potentially fatal human error.　性善説／～の教訓とする／人は必ず間違いを起こすという**性悪説**に立ち

Mr. B: If I may speak, I think we still need to motivate staff by giving them **more freedom or self-development** and by respecting their work.　自主性または自己研鑽

Mr. A: I agree on that. A regulation's **degree of severity** is based on the degree of danger that would result if the regulation were broken.　規則の**厳しさは**，それが破られたときに及ぼす危険の程度による

Mr. C: I would like to establish a safety regulation that impresses an MS to make sure he/ she doesn't **fall into some careless routine** which would endanger the patient.　不注意により患者を危険にさらすことのないような強制力を持つ安全基準

Mr. D: A QA program is **nothing but** doing things properly as a matter of fact. However, no matter how dedicated each staff is, this alone won't avoid potential errors.　品質保証とは当たり前のことを当たり前に行う，ただそれだけのこと

Mr. A: What do you mean by **"that's all there is to it?"**　ただそれだけのこと

Mr. D: Doing things properly is not always seen as proper from a **third person**'s point of view.　第三者の目からみれば

Moderator: OK. Let's confine ourselves first exclusively to problems on technique.

Mr. D: First, I'd like to point out the fact that most of us are not fully experienced with the machines newly assigned to us. Often we've had to change machines just when we finally get accustomed to one.

Mr. C: I don't think that quite **hits the nail on the head**. You know we have been doing our work using machines without any noticeable problems in our department until just the past two or three years.　当を得ているとは言えない

Moderator: You are violating the rules of brainstorming by criticizing somebody else's idea. One will hesitate to **come up with an idea** if the others **find fault with** everything he/she says. The statement "There is no knowing where the **effect** of an event will appear" **is never more true than** when applied to brainstorming. 意見を述べる／ケチをつける／"どんな結論が飛び出すかわからない"という成句［例えば、風が吹けば桶屋が儲かる：The wind blows (cause: 要因) and the bucket-makers finally make a profit (effect: **結果**)］／もっともだと痛感する

Mr. C: Oh, **I knew better**; but I just lost control of my tongs ..... 知ってはいたんですが、つい……

Moderator: OK. What was your idea, Mr. C?

Mr. C: I just want to say that if we have a section leader, sort of supervisor, in each section, careless errors will be reduced even under **trying conditions**. 習熟の課程でも

Mr. D: **There is something to that**, but the leader will **be tied up with** his / her own assignment. **The thing is**, we have a heavy workload. 一理はある／手がふさがっている／要は〜

Moderator: A work overload may be one of the causes of our trouble, but **leave it at that**. What else is there? 触れずにおく

Mr. A: My data tells us that the largest number of errors occur in emergency rooms and **special radiography rooms**. So I suggest that the MS in those rooms should remain there **no less than** one year. 特殊撮影室（例えば心血管造影室）／1年以上

Mr. B: Lack of basic knowledge of each expertise that **they should have** might be one of the problems, I'm afraid. They tend to **go for** only the newest technology, but I guess **that is the way it goes**. 身につけておくべき／飛びつく／仕方がない

Mr. D: Careless mistakes are not only due to mere carelessness, but also fatigue. I mentioned work overload again.

Moderator: Let's **straighten out** our idea up to this point. Mr. E, let me have a look at the **cause and effect diagram (Fig.1)**. As you know, Mr. E is an active member of the **in-house QA task force**. What are the items you wrote down? Well, lack of experience and orientation, overload that accompanies fatigue, thereby causing careless mistakes, and lack of basic knowledge. Now we can see **at a glance** that the primary cause is lack of experience with a machine due to the rapid **turnover** in assignments. I'll **relate** this conclusion **to** the hospital manager to have him take necessary measures.　整理する／特性要因図（fishbone diagram）／院内の品質管理対策委員会／一見して／頻繁な**勤務交代**／〜を〜に報告する（or, tell about 〜 to 〜）

Quiz
- **A.** Who brought up the brainstorming?
- **B.** Why does the hospital need to quickly set up some type of safety regulation in advance?
- **C.** How does Mr. A differentiate safety regulations from QA programs?
- **D.** Why does brainstorming generate a greater power than any one individual is capable of?
- **E.** Why isn't anybody allowed to criticize another's idea?

Answers
- **A.** Mr. A.
- **B.** Because lawsuits related to malpractice are becoming more common in Japan
- **C.** Safety regulations are based on a more serious belief that humans are by nature bad, that they will never be free from errors.
- **D.** Because one idea will lead to another person thinking up an idea, producing a synergistic effect or even a chain reaction
- **E.** One will hesitate to mention an idea if other members find fault with what he/she says.

Relevant expressions and additional phrases

1) Idiomatic phrases of debate　　ディベートの慣用表現
a) Making a claim　　主張する
1. We are very happy to take the **affirmative side** in today's debate and **urge** that 〜
   幸いにも**肯定側に立ち**／〜であることを**主張する**
2. We are **firmly convinced** that adoption of the resolution is urgent and inevitable.
   この仮定を採択することが急務であり，必須であると**固く信じる**
3. We **call for** adoption of the resolution.　　〜を求める
4. We urge rejection of the resolution.

b) Making refutation　　反論する
1. Let me refute each major argument in turn.
2. First of all, I found this difficult to believe.

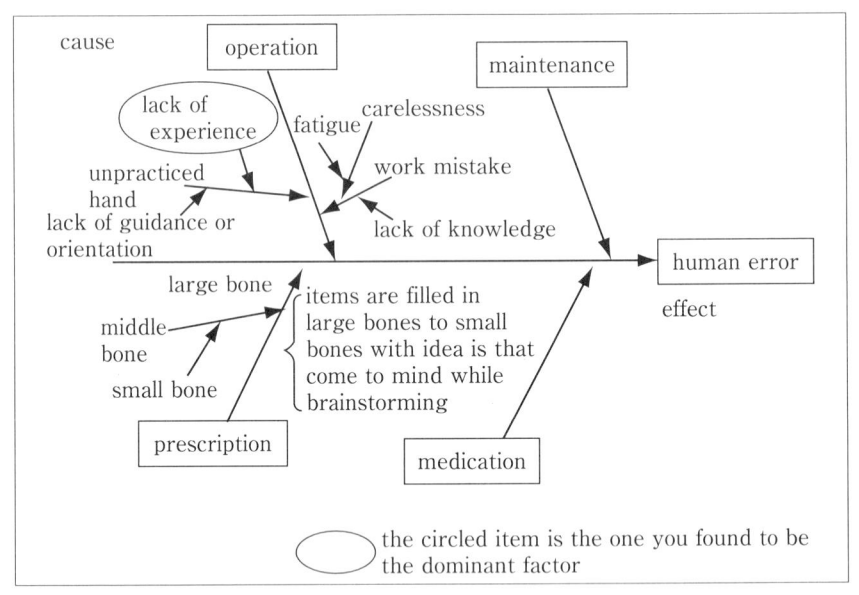

```
cause
        operation         maintenance
   lack of      carelessness
  experience  fatigue
  unpracticed      work mistake
  hand
  lack of guidance or   lack of knowledge        human error
  orientation
        large bone   items are filled in          effect
     middle         large bones to small
     bone           bones with idea is that
        small bone  come to mind while
                    brainstorming
        prescription    medication

              ⃝  the circled item is the one you found to be
                 the dominant factor
```

Fig.1 A branch of the cause and effect diagram for human error　　ヒューマンエラーの特性（effect）要因（cause）

3. Secondly, I think you have been **inconsistent**.　一貫性に欠ける
4. Finally, you have **failed to understand** the basic facts.　誤認がある
5. We of the affirmative position feel that the objections of the opposition are well thought out, but are not **persuasive**.　よく調べているが**説得力**がない
6. The affirmative side agrees that it is somewhat realistic, but **not what** we expect it **to be**.　期待に反する
7. It doesn't seem to me there would be any problem with that.
8. There is no scientific (**conclusive**) evidence to prove the opposing side's case. 反対側の論旨を支持する科学的（**決定的**）根拠が見当たらない

c) **Seeking clarification**　明快さを求める

1. What exactly did you mean by that?
2. Could you restate your point more clearly?
3. May I ask on what basis you say that?
4. Could you explain it in greater detail?　もう少し詳しく

d) Concluding statements   結論を述べる

   ① So, overall, the disadvantages of adopting the plan outweigh the advantages the affirmative side claims.

   ② On the basis of extensive research and investigation, it is my conclusion that this is the best and only measure available at present.

   ③ **In short**, it is clear that this argument is misleading.   つまり，その議論は間違っている

   ④ **In conclusion**, the plan of the affirmative side is bound to produce serious disadvantages.   結果として，肯定側のプランはきっと重大な不利益をもたらす

2) Idiomatic expressions of discussion   会議の慣用表現

a) Expressions of agreement   賛意表現

   ① You are exactly correct.

   ② I agree with you on that point.

   ③ We share the same view on that.

   ④ I was thinking the same thing.

   ⑤ I think you're quite right.

b) Expressions of disagreement   反対表明

   ① I can't go along with you on that point.

   ② I'm not sure if I agree with you on that ~

   ③ I almost agree with your opinion, but the trouble with it is that ~

   ④ That's not entirely correct.

   ⑤ I'm sorry, but I don't quite accept your reasoning.

c) Turning down a proposal   依頼を断る

   ① I'm afraid it would be impossible for me to ~ , but I appreciate your asking

   ② I wish I could...but thank you for asking anyhow.

   ③ I'd love to, but I can't.

   ④ We'd be rather reluctant to do that, unless ~   ~でなければその気になれない

d) Insisting on one's own opinion   自身の意見に固執する

   ① You've taken it the wrong way. My opinion is ~

   ② You may say so, but I think otherwise.

   ③ That's your opinion. What I think is ~

   ④ You're misinformed, and let me tell you why I think so.

e) Appealing to reasonableness   理論性の要求

① Wait a minute. What you said at the end seems to **contradict** what you said at the beginning.　言葉に**一貫性**がない
② I think you're **carrying** this **too far**.　極端に走る
③ Don't you think you are exaggerating a bit?
④ If you will listen a moment, I think you will see what I am trying to say.

f) **Identifying the key point**　要点の指摘
① What it comes down to is that ~　つまり，それは～
② The bottom line is ~　結局のところは～
③ To get straight to the point ~　端的に言えば～
④ The main point of what I have tried to say is ~

g) **Negotiation**　交渉
① We need a mutually satisfying compromise **worked out**.　お互いが満足するような妥協点を得るよう**努力する**
② **To this end**, we should not **hold back** any of our claims.　結論をみつけるために，遠慮なく主張し合う
③ We're **not getting anywhere** with our discussion deadlocked like this.　このまま対立したのではどうにもならない（cf. go around in a circle：堂々めぐりをする）
④ Well, I guess we **have no choice but to** accept it.　～せざるを得ない
⑤ Let's **leave** our minor differences **untouched** until later.　触れずにおく（cf. Minor differences must be submerged for the greater common interest：小異を捨てて大同につく）

3) Idiomatic expressions for general assembly　総会の慣用表現
a) **Approval of minutes**　議事録の承認
① Would you take a look at the **minutes** which have been delivered to each of you for reference?　お手元にお配りした**議事録**
② Are there any additional corrections to the minutes as read?
③ If not, the minutes **stand approved** as corrected.　このまま**承認された**
④ If there are not any further corrections, we will **move on to** today's agenda.　本日の議題に**移る**

b) **Proposal of motion**　動議の提出
① I would like to put a **motion** before the meeting.　**動議**を提出する
② I **move** the adoption of the resolution which we have proposed.　決議案を採択

していただくことを**提案する**
- ③ II propose a **motion** before the meeting.　　動議を提出する
- ④ I move to amend our code of conduct.

c) **Statements of Ayes and Nays**　　評決の表現
- ① I am in favor of this motion.　　動議に賛成
- ② I **second** the motion.　　動議に**賛成する**
- ③ I object to the motion.　　に反対する
- ④ I wish to have this motion withdrawn, **if I may ask**.　　できましたら，動議の撤回を

d) **Compromise proposal**　　妥協の依頼
- ① We **cannot get anywhere** insisting on each motion unless we compromise.　　妥協せずに，自分の提案だけに拘るとどうにもならない
- ② I move to **table** the question.　　一時棚上げすることを提案する
- ③ I move to **stand adjourned** for a while to think over this proposal　　案件をさらに検討するため，一時**閉会**を要求する

e) **Vote on motion**　　動議の評決
- ① I would like to **take a vote** on this proposal.　　本案について**評決をとる**
- ② Those in favor of the motion will say "Aye." And those opposed will say "Nay."
- ③ The motion's **carried** by an overwhelming majority (by a close vote).　　圧倒的多数（かろうじて）**可決された**
- ④ The **nays have it**, and the motion is dropped.　　反対多数につき，本案は否決

Exercises VI.

VI-1. Stand on either side of the proposition and express your opinion in English using as many given words below as possible or at least five of them. The certificate renewal is required every two years in America for medical staff after receiving a certain amount of credit points by attending some continuing education programs admitted by the professional organization.　　標記の提議に賛成，反対のどちらかの側に立ち英文で意見を述べなさい。免許更新制度とは，決められた時間の講習（continuing education）を受け，2年ごとに免許の更新をするものである。下記の"つなぎ言葉"や動詞句および副詞句を5つ以上含むこと（80 words or more）

Proposition 1. Registration for certificate renewal is necessary for medical staff.
Given words: 1) update their knowledge, 2) catch up with new technologies, 3)

demonstrates accountability to the public, 4) make a strong effort, 5) live up to, 6) fulfill their responsibility, 7) maintain competence, 8) professional obsolescence（技術面での遅れ）, 9) continuing education programs, 10) participating in, 11) renew the registration every two years, 12) end up, 13) consequently, 14) in other words, 15) in rality（実際は）, 16) avoid, 17) result in, 18) with regards to, 19) fall short of, 20) so to speak, 21) promotion based on seniority（年功序列）, 22) promotion on merits（成果主義）, 23) life-long employment（終身雇用制度）, 24) now that, 25) given that, 26) in that, 27) so that, 28) break down

FOR（賛成）／AGAINST（反対）
Circle either side you want to select (Opinions are not necessarily your own). どちらかを丸で囲む（本意である必要はない）

VI-2. Give your opinion in English for the proposition below. If necessary, use the following key phrases.

Proposition 2. Mercy killing (euthanasia) should be legalized.
論題2. 安楽死は合法化されるべきである

For: 1) the right of death with dignity rather than a painful and distressing death, 2) forced continuation of a vegetable state by extraordinary life-support equipment, 3) the true meaning of human life is based on individual will and awareness of one's own existence.

Against: 1) considered as a kind murder until new laws can clearly regulate euthanasia and lay down safeguards, 2) the law gives doctors and patients too much freedom, 3) further accelerates the trend toward underestimating the value of human life.

Example answerは巻末（付録の前）に掲載

Chapter VII.

International conference
国際会議

1. General session ——一般演題

Title: Smoking among Health Science University students in Japan
演題：日本の医療技術大学生の喫煙について

Chairperson:

Good morning ladies and gentlemen. Welcome to this session on epidemiology and health statistics. My name is Norio Saito. And I'm from The University of Daiwa Hospital, Tokyo, Japan. The co-chairperson this morning is Ms. Lee from Singapore General Hospital, Singapore. Before we begin, I would like to go **over** the rules.　ルールを（ざっと）**説明する**

Our session will be a series of presentations of short papers. Each presentation will be a maximum of ten minutes long. After eight minutes, there will be a green light to warn the speaker that there are two minutes remaining. At the end of ten minutes, you'll see a red light. Speakers who **go over** ten minutes will hear a buzzer. We hope it won't be necessary to use the buzzer. We have many speakers this morning, and want to save enough time for open discussion on any of the presentations at the end of the session.　10分**過ぎる**とブザーが鳴る

Okay, we'll **go ahead** now **with** the presentations and **begin with** the first one entitled "Smoking among Health Science University students in Japan" which will be presented by Mr. Morita from Japan. Mr. Morita, please.　を**始める**／から**始める**

Mr. Morita: Chairpersons, ladies and gentlemen. It's a great pleasure to be able to address you today. I'll be speaking on a study we conducted on smoking among university students of health sciences in Tokyo, Japan.

Introduction　緒言

The massive global increase in cigarette smoking over the last few decades is of major concern for public health internationally. The World Health Organization (WHO) has called tobacco **an emerging epidemic**. To combat this epidemic, evidence is needed on the **future health effects** of current smoking patterns, especially of **adolescents** among whom most smoking is initiated. Yet, little research has been done in Japan to document the patterns of adolescent smoking behavior. And even less information is available on medical-related students representing the next generation of health professionals and leaders. 一種の疫病／将来引き起こす結果／若者（未成年）

Subjects　目的

Accordingly, data for this study were collected over a 3-year period from **questionnaire surveys** of university students in the Schools of Nursing, Radiological Technology, Physical Therapy and Occupational Therapy. [This slide shows the total number of students for each school in the middle column and the number of students interviewed from each **school** in the right-hand column.] 口述アンケート／学科＠米国では学部（e.g. school of medicine：医学部）

Methods　方法

The study design was approved by an **advisory panel** containing independent researchers with experience in conducting surveys on smoking. Data were analyzed using the SPSS statistical software package and **significance** was presumed for probability $p < 0.05$. Analysis was done to determine any significant differences in questionnaire responses of students who were **current or ex-smokers** (ever smokers) and students who had never smoked (**never smokers**).　勧告委員会／優位差／現または既喫煙者／非喫煙者

Results　結果

Among the results, [as you can see in this slide,] significant differences between ever smokers and never smokers regarding **smoking perceptions** were apparent. More ever smokers thought cigarettes looked fashionable and helped communication. On the other hand, [as you can see here,] less ever smokers than never smokers thought smoking was an important health issue. Other issues this study **highlighted** included the increase in smoking among young females, underage smoking, the impact of **tobacco vending machines, peer modeling**, nicotine addiction, tobacco advertising, tobacco control education and **smoking cessation**.　喫煙に対する**考え方**／指摘する／タバコ自動販売機／同僚の模倣／禁煙

Conclusion　結論

In conclusion, I would like to say that these issues demand the attention of all of us, that their **ramifications** be discussed, recommendations made and measures taken for ensuring the health of our young people and future health professionals. Thank you for your kind attention.　結果が検討され，勧告ができ，対策が取られる

Quiz

- A. What is the major concern for public health that the speaker is talking about?
- B. What is the World Health Organization's view on tobacco?
- C. Among what age group is most smoking initiated?
- D. How and from where was the data for this research gathered?
- E. What issues concerning smoking were touched on in this survey?
- F. What kind of analysis was used in this study?

Answers

- A. The massive global increase in cigarette smoking over the last few decades
- B. The World Health Organization (WHO) has called tobacco an emerging epidemic.
- C. Adolescents
- D. It was collected over a 3-year period from questionnaire surveys of university students in Schools of Nursing, Radiological Technology, Physical Therapy and Occupational Therapy.
- E. Issues this study highlighted included the increase in smoking among young females, underage smoking, the impact of tobacco vending machines, peer modeling, nicotine addiction, tobacco advertising, tobacco control education and smoking cessation.
- F. Data was analyzed using the SPSS statistical software package and significance was presumed for probability $p < 0.05$. Analysis was done to determine any significant differences in questionnaire responses.

2. Special lecture ——特別公演
Title: Computer-Based Patient Records in Digital Hospitals
演題：デジタル病院における電子カルテ

Welcome to this special lecture of Computer-Based Patient Record in Digital Hospitals. It's a privilege for me to chair this session, and we are honored to have Dr. Frank as co-chairperson. In this session, three speakers from the University of Wisconsin Hospital (UWH) will give speeches in turn on **how** their **PACS**[*1] system **has progressed**. The first speaker is Dr. Cook, who will tell us the requirements of **RIS**[*2], the subsystem of the PACS system, taking **pediatric radiology** as an example. Then Mr. Haus will follow him to describe the hardware and software architecture of the RIS system. Finally, Dr. Kriz will speak about the **HIS**[*3]**-PACS integrated system, looking forward to** the future goal of filmless and paperless departments. Now, let's **start off with** Dr. Cook. **PACSの進展過程について**／小児放射線科／HIS-PACSの統合システム／フィルムや（医療・事務）用紙のいらない病院を**目指して**／**～から始める**

Dr. Cook:

What I'd like to do is discuss the operation of digital pediatric radiology. The software system which you'll hear mentioned by the name RIS, **stands for** Radiology Imaging System. This is the production system which the clinician actually uses in order to get patient images.　　～の略語である

In order for clinicians to perform diagnosis, they require some new digital images, but also require **historical images** from a patient's folder. These historical images are **brought in** with a **lazar digitizer**, which, looking at the average patient folder and what a patient needs our hospital, in general, we need to digitize three films per patient for each new patient that comes into our department.　　過去に撮影された画像／（コンピュータに）取り込まれた／レーザ収集デジタル化装置

If we save the computed radiography images in their original size, we would have 1,200 **megabytes** of storage per week. Concerning scanned film, if we scanned, say, at 1024 squared, we would have 300 megabytes; so you can see that, our weekly total can be **anywhere from** 2000 megabytes to around 3000 megabytes or three **gigabytes**.　　メガ（10^6）バイト／～から～の間のいずれかの値／ギガ（10^9）バイト

In summary, what we require in pediatric radiology is a hardware/software system able to handle images in numbers around 720 images per week, and to be able to store images at a maxim of about three gigabytes per week. Now, I'd then like to **turn the talk over**

to Mr. Haus who will tell us a bit about what the elements of RIS are, and go on to discuss the hardware/software architectures of the system. Mr. Haus.　〜に発表を譲る
Mr. Haus:

I'd like to **go over** the clinical system that we have at UWH called the RIS system. The majority of images that are acquired for this system originate from a **Computed Radiography** (CR) system. Approximately 80 percent of the images are by way of this system and image data from the CR system is automatically transferred into the RIS system by way of a custom-built interface port that we built at UWH as well as a console monitor program that signals when the CR images are being acquired.　（概略を）述べる／コンピュータ画像装置（デジタル画像装置とは区別される）@RISのなかのsystemは場合によっては冗長性を持たせる

Our images that **are queried** for storage are initially **acquired** on magnetic disk here and they're reformatted and entered into the RIS data base. Actually, we have a **hierarchical structure**[*4] that we developed at UWH consisting of a magnetic disk shown here, on-line and off-line magnetic optical disk storage, as well as image in real-time disk storage that we don't have **photograph showing**.　検索される／収納される／階層構造／フィルムによる観察（診断）

This is a hardware diagram of the RIS system. The **central controlling computer**[*5] is a SUN/XX (shown here). The **acquisition devices** consist of the CR system, the laser scanner as well as a CT, MRI and ultrasound which are interfaced into this system by way of a magnetic tape drive as well as a **digital communication network**.　LAN（local area network）の中の中心となるコンピュータ／画像収集装置／デジタル通信回線

The image is not clear enough to make a primary diagnosis on the **512 workstation**. So our first attempt was to use the workstation and **make a compromise** between the **field of view** and **display resolution**. This slide on your right shows one mode that the 512 display station can work in, namely using image data that is 2000 by 2000 having only a one-sixteenth field of view as defined by this **box cursor** here and showing this at full resolution on a monitor directly below that image. The workstation has been upgraded to 1024 by 1024 which will soon be replaced by a 1900 by 1900 display station.　512本の走査線テレビモニタを持つワークステーション（端末装置）／妥協する／関心領域／表示分解能／ボックス型カーソル

Well, that concludes the section on pediatric radiology of what was actually the first PACS module that we tried to develop at WUH. I only talked about a **separate PACS module** in our department. The next speaker will touch upon HIS[*6], a more integrated

PACS, that aims at handling all patients' **data** in all departments in a hospital. Thank you for your attention.　分散管理型PACSサブシステム／全患者のデータ（apostropheの位置に注意）

Dr. Kriz:

Electronic archiving in a hospital requires **terabytes** of storage, with a need of **rapid retrieval** of hospital data. Radiology data storage requirements are very large compared to other documental data. The large image storage requirements quickly exceed our ability to process, store and archive them. Our evaluation of the current and projected future data needs show that we will soon be generating about four terabyte's per year.　電子情報保存／テラ（10^{12}）バイト／迅速な検索

With this in mind, we began searching for a large image storage system. **Given** the problem **that** we had experienced with a "tape" archive we decided to try and follow the **rule of thumb** and use optical disks stored in a large jukebox. This idea was not realistic because we would need six optical jukeboxes per year, each of which has the capacity of 660 gigabytes with 12 drives. We need to store client data for five years or more.　過去の磁気テープによる保存には問題があることを経験したことがあるので，**経験則**に倣い，光ディスクをジュークボックス入れる方法を検討した

At the end of our search, we came to the conclusion that while tape has suffered in the past by having a reputation for being **less than robust**, tape today no longer stretches, or needs to be cleaned. It has a lifespan of 30 years that rivals optical disk systems. On the other hand, **RAID** (Redundant Array of Independent Disks) was chosen for a near-term storage to serve as a **cache** for all data including **DICOM** images and general data. Each type of data is managed automatically by it's own characteristics **once polices** for that data have been determined and set. This automated migration of data **to and from** tape upon demand is the key to this system. The ability to move data around on tape, **keeping** a patient's entire history **together**, is another major advantage of tape.　過去にはテープは**脆弱である**との悪評はあったが，今では伸びたりせず，クリーニングの必要性もなくなり／短期のデータ保存にはRAID（複数の光ディスクを配列した収納型ディスク）を**保存場所**に選び，そこにダイコム（DICOM：Digital Imaging and Communications in Medicine）規格の画像と一般データを保存する／**一度**データの特定と設定を行っていたなら，その特性に応じて自動的に管理される／要求に応じてデータが磁気テープ間を自動的に**移動する**ことはこのシステムの鍵である／患者一人一人の（apostropheの位置に注意）全ての履歴を**まとめて**テープ間を移動するのも大きな特長である

As we made the transition from a film-based to a film-less hospital, we realized there must be a painless and efficient migration of data from current technology to the next generation type when it's developed and released even by different PACS **vendors**. The approach that we are taking is to allow these functions to be provided by the RIS. As Mr. Haus has stated, once images are loaded on the **review stations** the physicians will **query** the RIS for all **unread** cases. The RIS then provides a list to the review software and the appropriate images are presented to the physician. フィルム依存から電子情報管理病院への移行期間であるので（前後の病院の内容が異なるので双方に冠詞を付ける），次世代PACS機種が異業者によって開発・市販されたにしても次世代へのスムーズな転換が可能でなければならない。／画像が閲覧ワークステーションに入力されたら医師はRISに未読影の症例を問い合わせる

We are now using PACS as HIS and **braking down traditional inter-departmental boundaries** for exchanging data, such as results of lab tests **on demand** when a radiologist is making a diagnosis at a reviewing station. He or she can get any information just by clicking an **image display button** on the report display window. PACSをHISとして用い，**部署間の情報交換の垣根を取り除く**／必要に応じて／レポート表示ウィンドウの**画像表示ボタン**をクリックするだけで

In the near future, the systems will span not only multiple departments but also medical institutes including **private clinics within the region**. In recent years, there are indications of an emerging architecture **paradigm shift**, a seamless shift to a new system architecture, in adopting **distributed object technology (CORBA)** for enterprise integration (**IHE**[*6]). For the time being, the **distributed computing** will be the main stream until a larger-scale **centralized control** system becomes available. The distributed computing is based upon the notion of an **Object Request Broker** (ORB) that is used to register objects and modes across a network and is accessed by **applications** at a **clinical workstation** wishing to utilize or modify information over the network. 地域医療施設／アーキテクチャーの**漸次移行**／CORBA（the Common Object Request Broker Architecture：分散オブジェクトシステム）／IHE: 医療企業間情報統合化／分散コンピューティング／集中管理システム／OBR：各目的・方式ごとに分散したシステム／アプリケーションソフト／臨床端末装置

Notes: *1 PACS （Picture Archiving and Communicating System）：画像保存・伝送システム，*2 RISはPACSのサブシステムで，放射線検査オーダリング，検査実施内容，診断レポート等を管理する，*3 HIS （Hospital Information System：病院情報システム）は放射線科中心のPACSの規模を病院全体に広げ，病歴，検査，処方，看護情報，物流，医療会計等を管理する，*4 各階層（レイヤ）から成り application layer を最上位とする．各レイア間のやりとりの規定がinterfaceである，＊5 中央制御コンピュータ：通常は異機種（heterogeneous）ネットワーク環境が主流であるので，LANによる複数のワークステーションを結んだ水平機能分散が行われ，その中心となるコンピュータを指す．イーサネット（Ethernet）はLAN間を結ぶプロトコルの一例である，＊6 IHE（Integrating the Healthcare Enterprise：医療企業間情報統合化）は，米国の医療機関は民営企業 Enterprise となったので，狭義にはHOM傘下の病院システムを指す（第6章　ディベート参照）．日本では，現況のIHE-Jは院内部署間の情報統合化が主体で，医療情報統合化とも訳される．

Quiz

Answer the following questions referring to the last part of Dr. Kriz's speech.
A. How is PACS different from HIS?
B. What does the word "architecture paradigm shift" mean?
C. Why is a distributed object system used for realizing HIE?
D. What does a physician access at a clinical workstation? Why?
E. Arrange the four computer systems, in the above questions, for obtaining digital images from the largest-scale system to its consecutive subsystems.

Answers

A. PACS is used only for radiological information but HIS is used across departments including documental data as well.
B. It is a gradual shift of computer architecture phasing out the conventional one while phasing in a new system.
C. Because current computer systems are wanting in capacity for treating huge data.
D. An Object Request Broker through which he or she can utilize or modify information over the network.
E. The order is HIS, PACS, RIS and a clinical workstation.

Relevant expressions and additional phrases

1) Tips for an effective power point presentation　　パワーポイント発表の要領

1. Present information relevant to audience.　　聴衆に適切な情報
2. Stay focused on the main topic.　　主題に的を絞る
3. Select slide colors that contrast and project well.

Chapter VII. International Conference 175

④ Choose a font size and style that is easy to read. (i.e. 28 point or more within 8 lines)
⑤ Minimize amount of text and type phrases rather than sentences.
（Bullet your information if possible）／箇条書きにする（i.e. itemize）
⑥ Make use of "spell check"and be sure to rehearse.　予行演習を丹念に
⑦ Employ graphs, charts and tables for summarizing data.
⑧ Add graphics, photos, sound, animation and resource links to enhance communication.
⑨ Don't **clutter** slides.　一枚のスライドに過剰な情報を入れないこと
⑩ Remember to thank the audience for their attention (at the end).

2) key expressions for powerpoint slide projection and room lighting　パワーポイントスライド発表と室内灯に関する重要表現

a) **Apologizing for a problem with a PowerPoint slide**　スライドの不手際を詫びる

① I'm sorry, my PC won't **boot** the system **up**. Wait a moment, please.　立ち上が（る）らない（cf. shut it down: 終了する）
② I'm sorry, my PC **froze**. Let me **reboot** (reset) it.　フリーズした／再起動させる（cf. Retrieve with **undo**, if you delete a slide by mistake再生させる）
③ Let me check **Projector Wizard** to see if the wizard actually doesn't connect my PC to the projector.　プロジェクタ自動選定機能
④ Will you, Sir, check if it **is plugged in**?　プラグがしっかり嵌っているか
⑤ Sorry, the slides are advancing rather fast. So I will remove the **automatic timer**.　スライド切り替え**時間設定**を解除する
⑥ I'm sorry you might not be able to see this graph clearly. So I'll zoom the **circled** key part. Let me switch to the film slide.　丸で囲んだ重要な部分を拡大する
　i.e. The laser pointer can serve for a mouse to point out or circle key areas of the slide.
　or, Let me click a pop-up menu so I can use a Pen to circle the key area each time.　ポップアップオプションからペンを選び，スライドに円をドラッグするとき
⑦ Could you please zoom the area...focus it a little better? It's still a little out of focus. That's it. Thank you.　プロジェクタ担当者に依頼するとき
⑧ I'm sorry. I just noticed this picture is backwards. let it be for the sake of tim　写真を反転させたいが時間がないとき

⑨ It appears I have been careless and **left out** a zero (**put** in an **extra zero**) here...here, where I'm pointing the arrow.　ゼロを1個入れ忘れた（余計に入れた）

⑩ Let me answer the question using another slide (**hidden slide**) I have on hand to support my answer.　予備のスライド（**非表示スライド**）を使用したい

⑪ Wait a moment please. I'll switch files from the slide to the movie.　スライドを動画ファイルに変える

⑫ In order to save time, I'll skip the next slide.

⑬ Because we are **short of time**, I'll **fast forward** until the desired slide is displayed.　時間が**なくなったので**，スライドを**早送りする**

b) Controling the room lighting　　室内灯の調整

① Could I have the lights dimmed, please?
② Dim the lights, please.
③ Darken the room a little more, please.
④ May I have the lights on?
⑤ Lights on, please.

3. Key expressions for the chairperson
——司会者のための重要表現

1) When time is running short　　時間が足りなくなってきたとき

① Mr. Morita, are you almost finished?
② Could you please hurry up a little, Mr. Morita?
③ Excuse me, Mr. Morita, but your time is up. Would you be so kind as to summarize your paper briefly?
④ Yes, but please be brief. (In response to the request, "May I just give my conclusion?")
⑤ I'm sorry, Mr. Morita. I think you've taken up a little too much time, but thank you.
⑥ People who have questions can perhaps see Mr. Morita afterwards. (when the chairperson has to interrupt a presentation that has gone overtime)

2) Idiomatic expressions in a pressing situation　　とっさのときの慣用表現

Normal expressions are put in blackest. [ ] 内は平常時の表現

① Try to move along. [Please keep going and get onto the next point.]

② We need to speed things up. [We need to move along more quickly.]
③ Could someone get the lights? [Would someone please turn out (turn on) the lights?]
④ We're out of time. [We have to stop now.]
⑤ Could you run that by me again? [I didn't understand what you said. Please explain it to me.]
⑥ I didn't get what you said about the first point. [I didn't understand what you meant when you were talking about the first point.]
⑦ Wrap thing up quickly, please. [Conclude your speech quickly, please]

3) When no one asks Mr. M a question　　M氏に対する質問がない場合
① Does anyone have any questions for Mr. M?
② Well, since no one seems willing to start asking questions, I'll ask one myself.
③ It looks as though the audience has understood you completely. Thank you, Mr. M.　演者に気まずい思いをさせないための表現

4. At a special speech　　――特別公演で
1) Introduction　　紹介

Dr. Smith, would you please come to the rostrum? It's my pleasure to **introduce to you Dr. Smith,** ladies and gentlemen. We are very happy to have Dr. Smith as our guest speaker this morning. Dr. Smith is so famous in our community that many of you probably know him better than I do. However, for the benefit of those who are unacquainted with Dr. Smith and his accomplishments, I would like to give a brief summary of the excellent work he has done in health sciences during the past five years.　語順に注意（public speechの場合）／cf. Let me introduce my colleague to you （informal）

2) Ending remarks　　終わりに

Thank you, Dr. Smith. That was an excellent speech. Your presentation will help us keep up with recent progress in this field, and we certainly wish you **continued health** and involvement as an international leader. Thank you very much.　変わらぬ健康を

3) Presentation of certificate along with a gift　　贈呈品と認証の授与

Chairperson (CP):　　Dr. Smith, will you please stay here for a minute? We are going to have a little ceremony. Please step to the center of the platform. **On**

	behalf of all our membership, it is my great pleasure to present you with this certificate commemorating the presentation of your lecture, along with this **small token of our esteem and our gratitude**.　〜を代表して／尊敬と感謝の意を添えてささやかな贈り物
Dr Smith:	Shall I open it now?
CP:	Please do. ＜or＞ You needn't. It has already been packaged for you to take home.

5. Key expressions for discussion periods
——質疑応答のための重要表現

1) Asking for questions from the floor　　会場からの質問を求める

① CP (Chairperson) : Let's now **proceed to** some questions or comments from the audience.

② If you have a question, please step to the nearest microphone, **identify** yourself, the country you represent, and the speaker to whom you would like to **direct** your question.

③ AUD (Audience) : Yes, may I, Mr. Chairman?

④ CP: Yes, sir (ma'am). Please use the microphone and identify yourself.

⑤ AUD: Can you hear me?

⑥ CP: No, sir (ma'am). The microphone **isn't working**. Please turn it on. ＜or＞ We can't hear you very clearly. Would you please **step closer to** the microphone?
　質疑応答に入る／自己紹介をする／質問を向ける／入っていない／〜に近づく

2) Asking for partial clarification　　ある部分の詳述を求める

Mr. X:	I would like to **ask** Mr. M a **question**. You mentioned that... Could you give us some more details on that?　　語順に注意 ask a question to Mr. M は誤り
Mr. M:	Yes, I'd be delighted to...

3) Making a comment rather than raising a question　　質問というよりコメントを述べる

Mr. X: 　I would like to raise a question about... The size determined by the method you used tends to be underestimated. On the other hand, the value measured by the method proposed by Mr. A is likely to be overestimated. Have you

Chapter VII. International Conference   179

	ever compared the results?
Mr. M:	No, we haven't tried that yet. It **would be** a good idea. Thank you.　そうかも**知れない**

4) Asking about a comparison   比較を尋ねる

① Mr. X: First let me compliment Mr. M on his innovative and provocative work. I'd like to ask you two questions. My first question is... The second one is, what do you think about...

② Mr. M: Would you be more specific about your first question?

③ Mr. X: What I meant to ask is...

④ Mr. M: ... May I have the second question repeated? I didn't quite understand it.

⑤ Mr. X: To put it simply...

⑥ Mr. M: I think that question could be better answered by Mr. S than by me.

5) Directing the question to another speaker   他の演者に質問を向ける

① Mr. X: This may seem like a rather **trivial question**, but would you mind telling me about this..., Mr. M?

② Mr. M: Actually, that's a **good question**...

③ CP: Mr. M, you're **getting off track** a bit. Please confine your remarks to Mr. X's question.

④ Mr. M: My apologies, Mr. Chairman. I **got carried away**.
つまらない質問／お答えしかねます（語調によっては度を越した質問に対する間接的な拒否ともなるのでニュアンスに注意：文字どおり**良い質問**の場合もある）／本筋から外れている

6) Asking for an answer with an example   具体例で答えてもらう

① Question: Excuse me, Mr. M, for interrupting. Could you please use an example to **illustrate** your answer?　はっきりさせる

② Answer1: Certainly. A good example is ... (formal)

③ Answer2: Sure. Let's suppose... (informal)

7) When you couldn't follow the question asked in English   質問を理解でないとき

① Question: If I understand correctly, you said that...

② Answer 1: I beg your pardon? (When you couldn't understand the question at all)
③ Answer 2: Are you asking whether I have compared our results with ones obtained by...... (This is confirming the question)
④ Answer 3: No, I didn't. But the reason is too complicated to explain in my limited English. May I answer your question later in private?
⑤ Answer 4: Let me answer the question first in Japanese, then Mr. Y will translate it into English. (When there's someone available to act as an interpreter)

6. key expressions for speeches at a party or dinner

——歓迎パーティ用のスピーチの重要表現

1) A conference officer gives a welcoming address　学会関係者による歓迎スピーチ

Good evening, ladies and gentlemen. My name is Mr. Tanaka, and I've been called upon to speak this evening. I'm not accustomed to speaking on such occasions, but as requested, I will say a few words. As one of the officers of this conference, I'd like to welcome all of you to the party tonight. I'd also like to give special thanks to the many participants from abroad who have traveled great distances to be here. We are very happy that all of you feel at home and hope you enjoy the party. Your visit here will help to promote friendship and deepen understanding among us. Thank you very much.

2) A participant gives an address in thanks　参加者の謝辞

I am speaking on behalf of all the participants, and in particular on behalf of those who have come from Singapore. I would like to thank President Suzuki and the Conference officers for inviting and welcoming us to this exciting party tonight. We thank you for the hospitality that you have extended to us throughout the Conference. I am sure all of us here will remember this event with fond and happy memories after our return home.

3) Acting as a toastmaster (toastmistress)　乾杯の音頭をあずかって

Ladies and gentlemen, I have the pleasant duty of acting as the toastmaster on this happy occasion. Glasses have been distributed to all of you. When everybody's ready, we'll call for a toast. I would like to propose a toast. Cheers!　では乾杯をしましょう。乾杯！

Exercise I. Pattern practice for useful expressions　文型練習

Complete the following sentences with the starting phrase followed by the given phrases in an interchangeable fashion.　出だしの文句（・）と下の網掛けの挿入句（◇）を交互に組み合わせて一つの文を完結させよ

1) Asking for a speaker's reasoning　理由を尋ねる

- For what reason do you believe that...　どんな理由で....と信じるのですか
- On what grounds do you believe that...　どんな根拠で....と信じるのですか
- What is your evidence that supports...　どんな証拠があって...とおっしゃるのか
- How do you account for the idea that...　どのような考えで....と言われるのかご説明ください

> ◇smoking is detrimental to the economy?　喫煙が経済に打撃を与える
> ◇smoking is a growing epidemic among young people?　喫煙が若者の間で蔓延している
> ◇health professionals aren't supportive enough of measures to curb smoking?　医療従事者は禁煙対策を十分に支持していない
> ◇Japan lags behind other industrialized countries in tobacco control measures?　日本は禁煙対策で他の先進国に劣る

2) Asking for possibility　可能性を尋ねる

- How long do you think it will be before...　あなたの考えでは...と言われるまでどれほどかかると思いますか
- What is your feeling about the possibility that...　あなたの...という可能性についてお聞かせください
- How great a promise is there that...　あなたは...ということについてどれほどの可能性があると思いますか
- To what extent has it evolved that...　どの程度...ということが進展していますか

> ◇we will replace all film viewing boxes with digital acquisition and display devices?　デジタル入出力装置がフィルム観察器に取って代わる
> ◇PACS will compete with the film-based system?　PACSがフィルム系に太刀打ちできる
> ◇the RIS module will provide radiologists access to data at clinical workstation?　RISモジュールにより，放射線科医が臨床端末装置で情報を得ら

◇the workstation will allow simple and quick review of digital images by acquiring patient's name or identification number?　端末装置で患者氏名やID番号を検索することで，デジタル画像の読影が簡単・迅速になる

3) Seeking confirmation　確認する

・If I understand your speech correctly, you meant that... Is that correct?　間違えなければ…と聞いていますが，その通りですか
・Did I understand you correctly to say that...　間違えなければ…と理解してよろしいですね
・I didn't quite get the last part of your speech. You mean that...　最後のところがどうもわからなかったのですが，…ということですか
・I'm sorry for this naive question, but I'm eager to know if...　未熟な質問で恐縮ですが，…というのかどうか非常に知りたいのですが

　　◇smoking is detrimental to the economy
　　◇smoking is a growing epidemic among young people
　　◇health professionals aren't supportive enough of measures to curb smoking
　　◇Japan lags behind other industrialized countries in tobacco control measures
　　　　　　　　　　　　〈 or 〉
　　◇the digital system can manipulate and reform film that is either overexposed or underexposed in to a useful range of densities (?)　デジタルシステムは露出過不足の写真でも読影可能な濃度に調整できる
　　◇once the disk is filled with data, an image can be retrieved in a reasonable amount of time (?)　ディスクに一度データを収納すると，画像の呼び出しは適度の速さだと
　　◇the chest radiograph generates at least 5M bytes, which means the optical disk can store only 500 sheets of film (?)　胸部写真はどうみても5メガバイトの情報があり，光ディスクはその500枚の写真しか収納できない
　　◇the image compression technique* will provide significant reduction in the number of data without compromising the quality of the clinical image (?)　画像圧縮技術で，診断価値を損なわずに十分にデータ数を減らせる
　　＊i.e. irreversible compression method：非可逆的圧縮法（収納枚数は一桁上げる）

4) Giving an opinion to a speaker　　コメントを述べる

・I completely agree with you that ...　　あなたの...という考えに全く賛成です。
・I think we all agree that...　　誰もが...ということには賛成のことと思います。
・I'm sorry, but I don't quite agree with your opinion. I understand that...　　あなたは...という意見でしょうが，残念ながら全く賛成というわけにはゆきません。
・What you said was right. I also feel that...　　その通りと思います。私も同様に...と思います。

The given phrases are the same as those in 3).　　挿入句は3)と同じものを使う

5) Asking for exactness　　正確さを尋ねる

・Have you had any experience with doing this in your research?　　あなたの研究でこのことを行ったことがありますか。
・Do you have any evidence to believe that?　　そう信じられる証拠がありますか。
・Do you have any data that would support such a policy?　　そのような方針を支持するデータをお持ちですか。
・Have you reached a conclusion on the cause of the problem?　　その問題の原因について結論を得ていますか。

　　◇My answer to your question is that...
　　◇As to your question, I would say that...　　あなたの質問に対する私の答えは...としかいえません
　　◇All I can say in answer to this question is that...　　あなたの質問についてお答えすれば，...としか言えません
　　◇I don't really have a good answer, except to say that　　答えになるかどうかわかりませんが，...と言うしかありません

The given phrases are the same as those in 3)again.　　指定の挿入句は3)と同じとする。

6) Seeking clarification　　明快さを求める

Substitute A with the given words.　　Aに指定語（◇）を入れよ。

・Will you elaborate on A?　　Aについてもう少し詳しく述べて
・Will you be more specific on A?　　Aについてもう少し具体的に
・Could you illustrate A more clearly?　　Aについてもっとわかりやすく
・Are you referring to A?　　Aのことをおっしゃっているのですか

　　　　◇quantity of memory（記憶容量）
　　　　◇image acquisition（画像収集）

◇image compression（画像圧縮）
◇patient's pictorial index（患者画像検索）

7) Asking for comparison　比較を尋ねる

Substitute A and/or B with the given words.　指定語A/B（◇）を入れよ

・How do you relate A to B?
・How do you compare A with B?
・What would you say are the differences between A and B?
・What is the main difference between A and B?
・AとBにはどのような関係があるのですか。

◇the access time / the transmission time
◇the PACS system / the RIS system
◇pixel number / scanning density
◇picture archiving / picture retrieving

Exercise II.　Japanese / English Drill

1. これであなたの質問の答えになったでしょうか。
2. パワーポイントスライドの試写はお済みになりましたか。
3. 英語の能力で**気が引ける**とか**恥ずかしい**と思うより、聴衆にわかってもらえるように努めなさい。そうするともっと**気が楽になります**。
4. 演者の皆さん、司会者を探しに**ここを離れない**ほうが良いですよ。**行き違いになる**といけませんから。
5. 次の演者の方は**次演者席**までお進みください。
6. 森田さん、**事務局本部**からお電話ですよ。
7. 少し時間が残っています。演者の方で今までのご発言に何か付け加えることがあるでしょうか。
8. 学会関係の方ですか。どこで予備用のスライドを返してもらえるのでしょうか。
9. **質疑応答**に同時通訳どころか、まったく通訳が予定されていないと聞いて**気が重く**なった。聞き取れないものをどう答えるのだろうか。
10. **国内委員会**で賛成された動議が、本会議で**公式**に満場一致で採択された。
11. この**運営委員会**は学術プログラムの進行に最新の注意を払っているばかりでなく、周辺サービスにも気を配っている。

Example answerは巻末（付録の前）に掲載

References
参照文献

Chapter I.

1） L. S. Torres: Basic Medical Techniques and Patient Care for Radiologic Technologists（fourth edition）. J. B. Lippincott Company, 1993.
2） 佐藤伸雄：放射線科における実践英会話改訂版．医療科学社，1990．
3） 高杉尚孝：NHK英語ビジネスワールド3月．日本放送出版協会，2002．

Chapter II.

1） The American National Red Cross: First Aid Responding to Emergencies. Mosby Year Book, 1991.
2） 東京消防庁救急部監：救急ワード・ブック．全国加除法令出版，1984．

Chapter III.

1） M. Smith: Diet and Cancer Connection. *Health Sciences*, **11**・4, 234〜242, 1995.
2） 富野康日巳・編：生活習慣病・基礎知識とセルフケアへのアプローチ．医学書院，2000．
3） 益尾　清：万病の引き金・活性酸素に負けない法．農文協，1998．
4） 板倉広重・他編：別冊NHK今日の健康・生活習慣病の医と食の辞典．日本放送出版協会，2000．
5） 森瀬春樹：体脂肪コントロールブック．株式会社 DHC, 2002．
6） 渡辺昌祐：うつ病と神経症（改訂増補版）．主婦の友社，2001．
7） 福原義春・他：美しく年を重ねるヒント．求龍堂，1998．
8） 佐藤伸雄：医療スタッフのための米会話．医療科学社（改訂版），2002．

Chapter IV.

1） A. Ehrlich：Medical Terminology for Health Professions（second edition）. Delmar Publishers Inc., 1993.
2） C. P. Anthony：G. A. Thibodeau; Structure & Function of the Body（seventh edition）. Times Mirror / Mosby College Publishing, 1984.
3） D. A. Woodrow：Introduction to Clinical Chemistry. Butterworths, 1987.

4) A. W. Currie：Basic Histology and Cytology. Churchill Livingstone, 1988.
5) 沖中重雄・他監：臨床雑誌内科．**61**・6（増大号），南江堂，1988.
6) 土屋俊夫・監：臨床検査の看護へのいかしかた．医歯薬出版，1989.
7) 山本敏行，鈴木泰三，他：新しい解剖生理学．南江堂，1997.
8) 鎌谷直之：尿酸値が高い人が読む本．主婦と生活社，2000.

Chapter V.

1) I. A. Kapandji：The Physiology of the Joints, Volume I, Upper Limb. Churchill Livingstone, 1993.
2) I. A. Kapandji：The Physiology of the Joints, Volume II, Lower Limb. Churchill Livingstone, 1987.
3) L. S. Lippert：Clinical Kinesiology for Physical Therapist Assistants（third edition）. F. A. Davis Company, 2000.
4) R. McRae：Clinical Orthopedic Examination（third edition）. Churchill Livingstone, 1990.
5) T. H. Berquist：Imaging of Orthopedic Trauma（second edition）. Raven Press, 1992.
6) P. W. Ballinger：Merrill's Atlas of Radiographic Positions and Radiologic Procedures. Volume I（seventh edition），Mosby Year Book, 1986.
7) L. Peterson, P. Renstrom：Sports Injuries；Their Prevention and Treatment. Mosby Year Book, 1986.
8) 井原秀俊，中山彰一・他：図解―関節・運動器の機能解剖―上肢・脊柱編．協同医書出版社，1984.
9) 井原秀俊，中山彰一・他：図解―関節・運動器の機能解剖―下肢編．協同医書出版社，1984.
10) 廣島和夫，米延策雄：これでわかる整形外科X線計測（改訂第2版），金原出版，1993.
11) 岩谷　力，佐直信彦・他：運動障害のリハビリテーション．南江堂，2002.
12) 堀尾重治：骨・関節X線写真の撮りかたと見かた．医学書院，1992.

Chapter VI.

1) N. Sato：Japanese RTs Struggle for Professional Status. *Radiologic Technology*, **64**, 319～320, 1993.
2) J. V. Valkenburg：Brian Lopatofsky and others, The Role of the Physician Exten-

der in Radiology. *Radiologic Technology*, **72**, 45〜50, 2001.
3) R. M. Friedenberg：The Role of the Supertechnologist. *Radiology*, **215**, 630〜633, 2000.
4) Annual Report to Registered Technologists：Continuing Education Requirements for Renewal of Registration of the American Registry of Radiologic Technologists. April, 8〜17, 1997.
5) K. Duke：Corporate Compliance Programs, Framework and Implementation. Proceedings of AHRA 26th Annual Meeting & Exposition, 1998.
6) K. Ishikawa：What is Total Quality Control? The Japanese Way. Prentice-Hall, Inc., 1985.
7) 今野　洋：ディベート教室・実践編―事例研究．学書房，1983．
8) 岩下　貢：ディベート言論・総合編．学書房，1983．
9) 廣瀬輝夫：日本よ！　米国医療を見習うな．日本医療企画，2000．
10) 田村　誠：マネジドケアで医療はどう変わるか．医学書院，1999．
11) 佐藤伸雄：米国における放射線技師免許の更新制度．*Innervision*, **4**, 68〜69, 1998．
12) 佐藤伸雄：医療スタッフのための米会話（改訂版）．医療科学社，2002．
13) 佐藤伸雄：放射線科における実践英会話（改訂版）．医療科学社，1990．

Chapter VII.
1) M. Smith：Smoking among students of allied health sciences in Japan, Asia-Pacific Journal of Public Health, **12**・1, 17〜21, 2000.
2) S. Wong, M. Sullivan, et. al.: Net Generation Information Infrastructure for Digital Hospitals. Proceedings of the 12th International Symposium and Exhibition of CAR'98, 349〜353, 1998.
3) L. Acklen：Teach Yourself Microsoft Office 2000. SAMS, 1999.
4) 宮坂和男：私の考える画像管理システムの将来．新医療，**8**, 72〜74, 2002．
5) 蓮尾金博，高橋直幹：HISと連携したRIS・PACS・レポーティングシステムの構築．新医療，**8**, 86〜89, 2002．
6) 佐藤伸雄：放射線科における実践英会話（改訂版）．医療科学社，1990．

Example answer

Chapter. I

Concerning patient care, **the first thing to do** is make a great effort to build rapport with a patient. No matter how good one's technique may be, lack of cooperation from a patient may **result in** poor quality service. A good example of **building rapport** would be to smile at a patient and give him/her a clear explanation of the procedure prior to an examination. **As a result**, the patient can be more relaxed and well-prepared. **The last thing we want to do** is **fall short of** a patient's expectations by neglecting our clinical responsibilities or ethical considerations. We must maintain confidentiality of a patient's information and be sure that the patient has given informed consent to any procedure. **In other words**, we must **live up to** the confidence a patient places in us.

Chapter. II
II-1

Any person should know what to do in an emergency before medical help arrives, much less medical staff. They should have the ability to recognize emergencies and how to respond expediently. If you, as a medical staff, are the first responder to an emergency, you need to be able to make appropriate decisions regarding first aid care and take charge among passersby for coordinating response efforts. You can provide appropriate care and have confidence in your ability to respond to emergencies only when you have taken a course in first aid for CPR and Heimlic maneuver. If you have done nothing about learning first aid, you are at risk of encountering an emergency situation in which you are unable to respond professionally, resulting in possible loss of life and disgrace to your medical profession.

II-2

Good Samaritan laws（よきサマリア人法）とは，ひとりの男が旅の途中に道端にいた旅人を助けたという聖書のなかの有名な寓話に基づくものである。これは（米国の）州法で，一般市民や医療従事者を法的に守る（法的免除）ために制定された。誰もが自分の州でこの法の保護の下にあるか知らなければならない。もし救急現場に遭遇し適切

かつ慎重に対応したとき，Good Samaritan laws が結果を問わずに適用される。しかし，救助者は自分の修得能力の範囲を逸脱してはいけない。救助者は踏み込んだケアをする場合には，少なくともA，B，C（気道，呼吸，脈拍）を確認すべきである。はじめに専門家に援助依頼の電話をし，その上意識のある犠牲者からは（援助の）承諾を得ることを決して忘れてはいけない。

Chapter. III
III-1

Everybody knows that smoking is harmful to health since it causes several diseases, especially lung cancer. Furthermore, second-hand smoke can endanger persons around a smoker. Medical staff stand in a position where they must persuade the smoker, whoever it may be, to quit smoking. Who, though, can convince a patient that smoking is dangerous when he himself is smoking? Once we have chosen to become medical staff, we who smoke should stop smoking immediately to demonstrate accountability to the public.

喫煙はいろいろな病気，特に肺がんを誘発する原因となり，健康に有害であることは誰でも知っている。さらに，副流煙は喫煙者の周りの人々に危険を及ぼすおそれがある。医療人は，それが誰であろうと，喫煙者に禁煙を説得しなければならない立場にある。だが，自分自身が喫煙者であれば，誰が喫煙の危険を患者に納得させることができるだろうか。医療人になると決めたからには，社会に対して責任を全うするため，われわれ仲間の間でタバコを吸う者はただちに禁煙すべきである。

III-2

スーパーオキサイドリダクターゼ（SOR）で代表される活性酸素は，ある電子軌道に不対電子を持ち，それが他の原子から電子を奪い取ろうとしている酸素と定義される。この現象は酸化反応ともいわれ，この逆反応が還元反応である。SOR を消去するためにSOD（スーパーオキシド・デスムターゼ）と呼ばれる酵素がはたらき，大部分の SOR を過酸化水素に変え，次々と他の酵素が過酸化水素を消去していくが，いくらかは残ってしまう。この残りが細胞のなかの銅イオンや鉄イオンと結合して反応を起こし，ヒドロラジカルに変わる。最終的には，最初に発生した SOR と反応して最も毒性の強い一重項酸素に変身する。要約すれば，フリーラジカル反応とは酸化反応と言ったほうがよいかもしれない。それは単に，不対電子が軌道電子を埋めるために他の殻から電子を奪うものであるから（**Fig.3** の SOR 参照），軌道に電子がまったくない場合にはその反応はさらに激しくなる（**Fig.2** の一重項酸素を参照）。

Chapter. IV
IV-1
The role of HDL in **coronary heart disease** is protective rather than causative, as it combines with excess cholesterol and transports it to the liver, where it is metabolized and removed from circulation. That is why HDL is so called "**good cholesterol**", as opposed to LDH which is the most causative factor of **arterial sclerosis**.

IV-2
健常人では，すべての体液はホメオスタシス，すなわち体液平衡が保たれている。たとえば，体内の水分量は，水分の摂取量と尿排出量がほぼ等しく保たれる。体液のバランスが崩れると，脱水症や過水症になるのみならず，血中の電解質の濃度バランスも崩れる。電解質は溶液に解離して正の電荷（カチオン）とクロールのような負の電荷（アニオン）に分かれる化合物である。重要な正電荷としては，ナトリウム，カルシウムやカリウム等がある。

腎臓は電解質の主な調節機能を司るので，電解質のバランスが崩れると腎機能の異常を疑う。体液の酸塩基平衡も腎機能の指標となる。これは体液の水素イオン濃度pH（ピーエイチ）で表示する。 具体的には，pH=7で活性が正常，あるいは中和であり，血液は酸性でもアルカリ性でもない。腎臓はpHの恒常性を保つ重要の臓器である。 腎尿細管は血液から過剰な酸を取り除き塩酸基平衡を保つ。ただし，尿は排尿までに酸化されるので，尿のpH値は血液のpH値より1か2ほど低い酸性を示す。

IV-3
Every person knows smoking and excessive drinking is bad for health. I would like to focus on **obesity** that may develop into all kinds of lifestyle diseases. Obesity results from an over-intake of energy that cannot be consumed by the body, so that the surplus energy accumulates in adipose tissue or internal organs as fat. **Hyperlipidemia** is the most common result stemming from obesity and can develop dangerous complications, such as coronary heart disease and **arterial sclerosis**.

To begin with, it is important that one maintains a simple formula for effective weight control by being temperate in eating, yet partake of well-balanced nutrients. If you are aware of something lacking in nutrients, never hasten to depend on health **supplements** for the deficit. Instead, try eating some vegetables to help supply the deficit and maintain a good nutritional balance. Also, avoid a high intake of biased nutrients that inversely affect one's health.

Secondly, I recommend a person do **aerobic exercise** because lack of exercise brings about obesity. An obese person becomes a possible diabetic candidate due to lingering hyperlipidemia. Aerobic exercise, so-called "air-walking which lets one smile" or jogging are common examples of good exercise since they are moderate and sustainable exercises which can be carried out in daily life.

Chapter. V
V-1

Among medical health professionals, RTs are the only experts in the production of diagnostic images and in a key position for ensuring radiation protection for the patient. However, desired care may not be provided for the patient with their skill and care alone, since they are not familiar with skeletal muscles which usually don't appear on an x-ray image. On the other hand, PTs are specialists for rehabilitation with a deep knowledge of how to manage patients after surgical operations or injuries. They are good at patient transfer and lifting procedures knowing well the limit of a patient's ability to bear weight and how to position themselves to help brace a patient's weak side in the case of a fracture. They also know how to sit a patient from a reclining position, or lay him or her down on either side to turn to the supine position with the knees flexed. While both types of professionals are not in a position to take vital signs, and a nurse may be summoned to perform the task in an emergency situation, they must take responsibility for proper and efficient patient care. To avoid any technical interruption in their work, they must share knowledge beyond the area which they are trained, that is, they need to possess multidisciplinary knowledge. For effective team medicine, medical staff must have close contact with each other for each patient.

V-2

It is essential for aerobic walking to take broad steps with your forward foot pointed up and landing on the heal. Walk as fast as possible on an imaginary straight line with the back leg straight and striking the ground forcefully. As for a gait appearance, throw out your chest and extend your back with your head facing straight; but draw in the chin a bit so that you can look forward with the eye level directed a bit downward. Swing your arms widely to a point that the elbow bends at a right angle at the end of the arm swing (**Fig. 42**).

V-3

医学の進歩にともない，医師や異分野の専門医療スタッフが医療チームを組んで，個々の患者のニーズに対処することが求められる。これはチーム医療として知られており，スムーズで有効的なケアの実施にあたっては，各チームメンバーは学際的な知識や技能をもたなければならない。このチーム医療により，メンバー間に重要な情報の共有や密接な協調関係が生まれる。**決して忘れてはならないことは**，患者もチーム医療の一員であるということである。患者の協力や積極的な参加意識がないと，折角の医療従事者の努力が**無駄**になるおそれがある。

Chapter. VI
VI-1

For: Modern technology is so rapidly improving that registration for certificate renewal has become necessary for medical staff. They should **make a strong effort** to **catch up with new technologies** and **avoid professional obsolescence**. They need **to renew the registration every two years** after accumulating the necessary credit points earned by **participating in continuing education programs**. By doing so, they can **maintain competence** and **fulfill their responsibility. In other words**, they can **live up to** the patient's expectations, which will **result in demonstrating accountability to the public**.

Against: **Now that** the **life-long employment system** is **breaking down** in Japan, medical staff know that they cannot expect any **promotion based on seniority**. **With regard to** their promotion, only those who **update their knowledge** and maintain competence can expect a higher position, **so to speak, promotion based on merits**. Others will **end up** staying in the same position for the rest of their career, **given that** they make no effort towards self-improvement. **Consequently**, they will compete with each other **so that** they can survive in a race for promotion. I think that the mandatory renewal system is not necessary, **given that** a natural competitive system exists.

VI-2

I am against legalizing euthanasia / assisted suicide for the following reasons. To me, a request for assisted suicide is typically a **cry for help**. It is **in reality** a **call for** counseling, assistance, and positive alternatives as solutions for very real problems. Secondly, suicidal intent is typically **transient**. Of those who attempt suicide but are stopped, less than 4 percent **go on** to kill themselves in the next five years; less than 11 percent will commit suicide over the next 35 years.　　命嘆願／実際は〜を求めている／発作的／自殺未遂者のうち，実際に自殺をしたのは

Thirdly, terminally ill patients who desire death are depressed and depression is treatable in those with terminal illness. In one study, of the 24 percent of terminally ill patients who desired death, all had clinical depression. Fourthly, pain is controllable. Modern medicine has the ability to control pain. A person who seeks to kill him or herself to avoid pain does not need legalized assisted suicide but a doctor better trained in alleviating pain. Fifthly, in the U.S. legalizing **voluntary active euthanasia** [assisted suicide] means legalizing nonvoluntary euthanasia. State courts have **ruled time and again** that if competent people have a right, the Equal Protection Clause of the United States Constitution's Fourteenth Amendment requires that incompetent people be "given" the same "right."　　自発的安楽死を合法化することは非自発的安楽死も合法化する／複数の州裁判所が，何度も採決したことは，もしある人が該当するのであれば，合衆国憲法第14修正案，平等保護条例により，対象外の人も同じ権利を持つことになるということである

In the Netherlands, legalizing voluntary assisted suicide for those with terminal illness has spread to include nonvoluntary euthanasia for many who don't have a terminal illness. Half the killings in the Netherlands are now nonvoluntary, and the problems for which **"death in now the legal solution"** include such things as mental illness, permanent disability, and even simple old age. Finally, you don't solve problems by **getting rid of** the people to whom the problems happen. The more difficult but humane solution to human suffering is to **address** the problem itself.　　そのようなことから，現在の"合法的な解決による死"がもたらす問題は，…それに単に老齢であることをも含むことである／問題が生じる対象者を除外したのでは問題解決とならない／苦しみに対する最も困難で人道的な解決法とは（本人とその周囲の人々が）真正面から現実に立ち向かうことである

@ 動詞 address は confront とか deal with に置き換えられる。

Chapter. VII

1. Could that be an answer to your question?
 ⟨or⟩ Is that what you are asking for?
2. Have you already given a preview of your PowerPoint presentation?
3. Try to focus on making the audience understand you clearly rather than allowing yourself to **feel small** or **feel shy** about your English ability. This should help you **feel more relieved**.
4. Any of the speakers would **be better off not to leave here** to try to find the chairperson. You may **unknowingly cross paths**[*1].
5. The next speaker should proceed to sit in the **specially designated chair**.
6. Mr. Morita, you are wanted on the telephone in the **headquarters of the secretariat**.
7. We have only a short time left. Would any of you speakers like to add something to the speeches you've completed?
8. Aren't you a **conference officer**? Where can I go to **get** my backup-slides **back**?
9. I'm a little **concerned** to hear that no translation, **much less** simultaneous translation[*2], is planned for the **question-and-answer period**. How can I answer questions in English which can't be understood?
10. The **motion** which we **had seconded** in the domestic committee meeting **was** officially **carried** with a **unanimous** decision at the **plenary session**.
11. The **steering committee** works carefully to conduct scientific programs. **On top of that**, they handle **logistical** considerations[*3].

Notes: *1 i.e. miss each other, *2 cf. consecutive translation/逐次通訳　shadowing translation/順同時通訳（演者よりやや遅れる通訳), *3 (e.g. accommodation, traffic, lunch, etc)

@ Backup-slides are conventional film slides used in the event that the PC doesn't work.

Appendix 1

ANATOMICAL TERMS

解剖用語

1. **Anatomic Projections and Depressions**　突起と陥凹

Projections（突起）：側方にまたは母体構造より突出した突起（process）の総称で，下記の用語で分類される

 protuberance or process（隆起または突起）突出の一般用語
 tubercle（結節）小さな，円形の突起
 tuberosity（粗面）大きな，円形の突起
 trochanter（転子）大腿骨頚部の下部にある2つの大きな円形の突起で，大（greater or major）または小（lesser or minor）のいずれかで形容される
 condyle（顆）四肢関節部の円形突起
 epicondyle（上顆）顆の上部突起
 head（骨頭）長骨の上端
 coracoid or coronoid process（烏口（うこう）／鉤状（こうじょう）突起）くちばし状の突起
 malleolus（果）踵関節の両側にある棍棒状突起
 styloid process（茎状突起）長い，とがった突起
 spine（棘）鋭い突起
 crest（稜）稜線状の突起
 facet（小関節面）小さな，滑らかな表面をした関節突起

Depressions（陥凹）：空洞あるいは陥凹部のことで，次の用語で定義される

 groove（溝）浅い直線状の陥凹　e.g. interventricular g.：心室間溝
 fissure（裂）cleft またはgroove ともいう　e.g. superior orbital f.：上眼窩裂
 sulcus（溝）溝，堀または裂状陥凹　e.g. aortic s.：大動脈溝
 fossa（窩）穴，杯状陥凹，または空洞　e.g. coronoid f.：烏啄窩
 foramen（孔）血管，神経の通る骨の中の穴　e.g. alveolar f.：歯槽孔
 sinus（洞）くぼみ，溝，または空洞
  頭蓋骨内表面の血脈洞　e.g. cranial s.：頭蓋上脈洞
  副鼻腔として骨の中の空気洞　e.g. ethmoid s.：篩骨洞

2. **Part Locations and Positions**　部位および方向
　　anterior and ventral（前および腹側の）身体または臓器の前面をさす。足の前面の場合はdorsumまたはdorsal surface（背面）という
　　posterior and dorsal（後および背側の）身体または臓器の裏面を示す。足の裏面はplantar surface（足底）という
　　superior, cranial and cephalic（上，頭蓋および頭側の）身体の上方向をさす
　　inferior and caudal（下および尾側の）身体の下方向をさす
　　medial and mesial（内側および近心の）身体の正中または中心部，側方の反対
　　lateral（外側の）正中または中心部より離れる方向，左側・右側
　　central（中心の）臓器の中心部または主要部
　　peripheral（末梢の）臓器の末端部
　　internal（中心の）体，臓器の深部または中心部
　　external（外側の）表面で，周辺または最外側の部位
　　proximal（近位の）目的部への近傍，または組織の起始部
　　distal（遠位の）目的部から隔れた部位
　　parietal（壁在の）空洞の壁　e.g. p. anterior：前壁（胃または腔の）
　　visceral（内臓の）腔内臓器に用いられる　e.g. v. cavity：内臓腔

3. **Body Positions**　体位
　　supine（背臥位の），prone（腹臥位の），recumbent or decubitus（臥位の），dorsal recumbent ＝ supine（背臥位の），ventral recumbent ＝ prone（腹臥位の），lateral recumbent（側臥位の）
　　supinate（回外する）手のひらが上を向くよう前腕を回転させること
　　pronate（回内する）手のひらが下を向くよう前腕を回転させること
　　eversion（外反）外側に向くこと　e.g. e. of planter surface：足底部の外返し
　　inversion（内反）内側に向くこと　e.g. i. of vajina：膣内反
　　flexion（屈曲）2本の近接する骨に狭まる角度が小さくなるような関節の動き，または前屈，伸展と逆の動き
　　extension（伸展）関節を伸ばすこと，ある部分を伸ばすこと，または背屈，屈曲の逆の動き
　　abduction（外転）ある部分が体中心軸より遠ざかる動き
　　adduction（内転）ある部分が体中心軸の方向に向かう動き
　　decubitus（ディキュビタス）臥位となることを目的とした動きまたは体位。
　　＠Radiographyのdecubitusは水平X線束撮影

Appendix

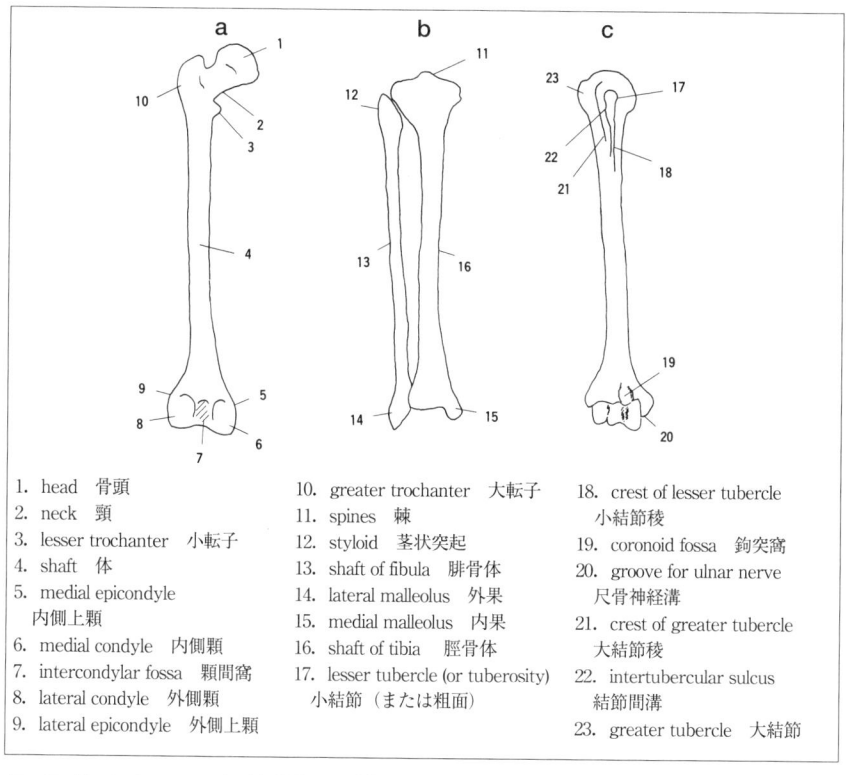

1. head　骨頭
2. neck　頸
3. lesser trochanter　小転子
4. shaft　体
5. medial epicondyle
　　内側上顆
6. medial condyle　内側顆
7. intercondylar fossa　顆間窩
8. lateral condyle　外側顆
9. lateral epicondyle　外側上顆
10. greater trochanter　大転子
11. spines　棘
12. styloid　茎状突起
13. shaft of fibula　腓骨体
14. lateral malleolus　外果
15. medial malleolus　内果
16. shaft of tibia　脛骨体
17. lesser tubercle (or tuberosity)
　　小結節（または粗面）
18. crest of lesser tubercle
　　小結節稜
19. coronoid fossa　鉤突窩
20. groove for ulnar nerve
　　尺骨神経溝
21. crest of greater tubercle
　　大結節稜
22. intertubercular sulcus
　　結節間溝
23. greater tubercle　大結節

Fig. 1　Posterior aspect of left femur (a) and anterior aspect of right lower leg (b),
　　　　Anterior aspect of right humerus(c)
　　　　左大腿骨の後面（a）と右下大腿骨の前面（b）右上腕骨の前面（c）

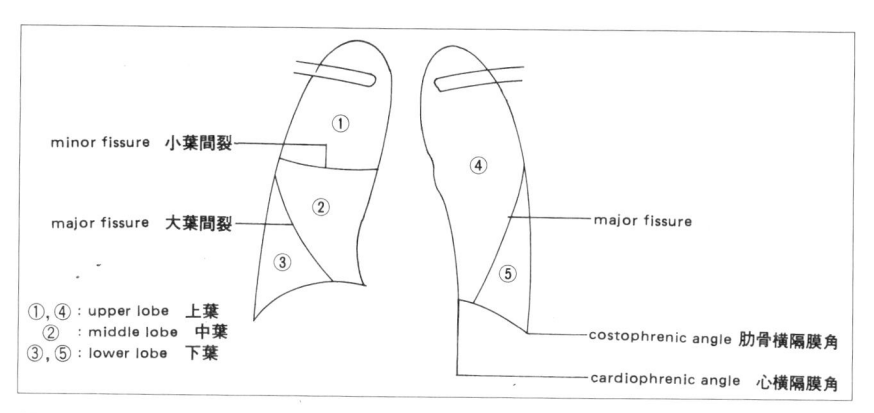

minor fissure　小葉間裂
major fissure　大葉間裂
major fissure
costophrenic angle　肋骨横隔膜角
cardiophrenic angle　心横隔膜角

①, ④ : upper lobe　上葉
② : middle lobe　中葉
③, ⑤ : lower lobe　下葉

Fig. 2　Lobes and interlobular fissures of the lung　肺葉と葉間裂

Appendix 2
ANATOMICAL AND COMMON NAMES FOR PARTS OF THE BODY
人体各部の解剖学的名称と一般名

Anatomical Term：解剖学的名称	**Common Name**：一般名
Head & neck 頭頸部	
1. mandible 下顎	jaw
2. thyroid cartilage 甲状軟骨	Adam's apple
3. neck 頸	throat
Anterior thorax 胸部（正面）	
4. clavicle 鎖骨	collarbone
5. sternum 胸骨	breastbone
6. thoracic area 胸部	chest
Upper extremity 上肢	
7. axilla 腋窩	armpit
8. humerus 上腕	arm
9. radius and ulna 橈骨・尺骨	forearm
10. carpal bones 手根骨	wrist
11. metacarpal bones 中手骨	hand
12. first digit 第1指	thumb
13. second digit 第2指	index finger
14. third digit 第3指	middle finger
15. fourth digit 第4指	ring finger
16. fifth digit 第5指	little finger（pinky or baby）
Abdomen 腹部	
17. any area of the abdomen 腹部の総称	stomach
18. epigastric area 心窩部	pit of the stomach
19. umbilical area 臍部	belly or tummy
20. hypogastric area 下腹部	lower stomach
21. hypochondriac area 心気部	flank

22. level of the third lumbar vertebra　第3腰椎高部　　waist
23. umbilicus　臍　　belly button or navel

Lower extremity　下肢

24. iliac crest　腸骨稜　　hip
25. subinguinal area　鼠径下部　　groin
26. greater trochanter　大転子　　hip
27. femur　大腿骨　　thigh
28. patella　膝蓋骨　　kneecap
29. tibia and fibula　脛骨・腓骨　　leg
30. metatarsus　中足（骨）　　foot
31. first toe　第1趾　　great or big toe
32. fifth toe　第5趾　　little or baby toe

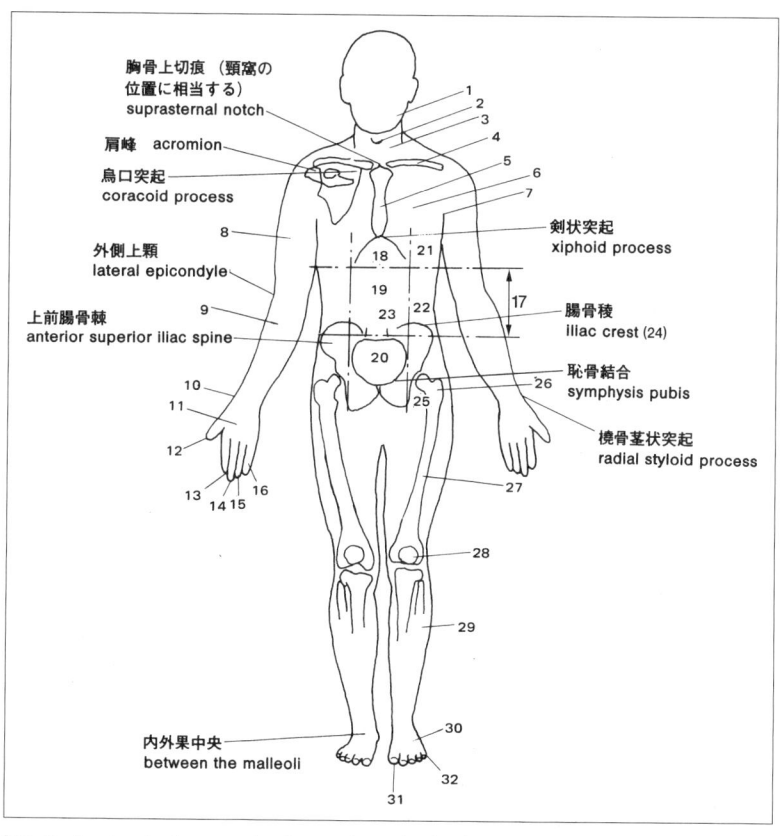

Fig. 3　Anatomical names for the parts of the body

4. Motions of Body Parts　体部の動き

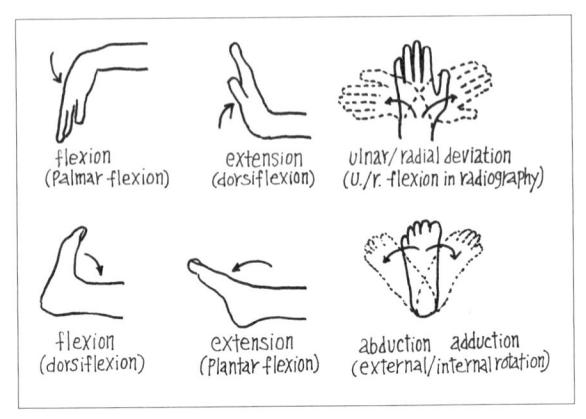

Fig. 4　Motions of hand and foot
　　　palmar flexion：掌屈, dorsiflexion：背屈, ulnar /
　　　radial deviation：尺屈／撓屈, plantar flexion：底屈

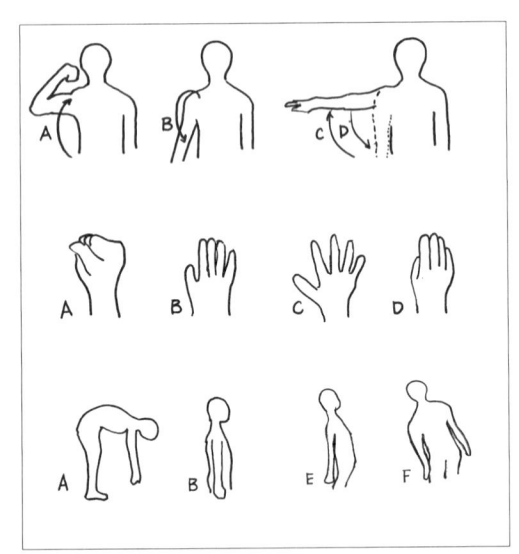

Fig. 5　Motions of upper extremity (upper), hand (middle) and trunk (bottom)
　　　A: flexion, B: extension, C. abduction, D: adduction, E: hyperextension（過伸展）, F: lateral bending（側屈）

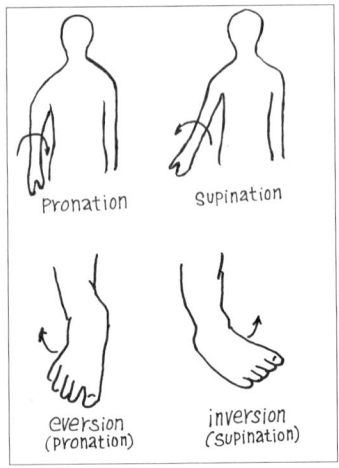

Fig. 6　Motions of forearm and foot

Appendix

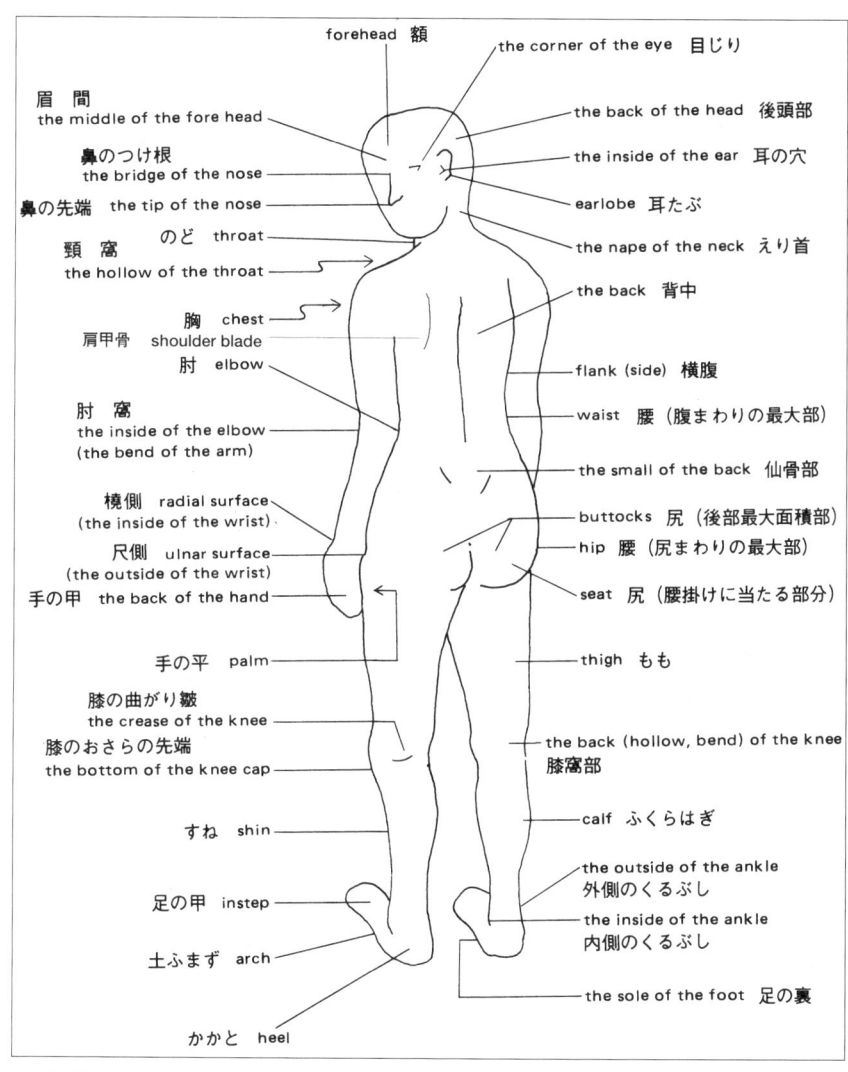

```
                    forehead 額
眉　間                         the corner of the eye　目じり
the middle of the fore head
                              the back of the head　後頭部
鼻のつけ根
the bridge of the nose        the inside of the ear　耳の穴
鼻の先端　the tip of the nose
                              earlobe　耳たぶ
頸窩　のど　throat
the hollow of the throat      the nape of the neck　えり首

           胸　chest           the back　背中
肩甲骨　shoulder blade
           肘　elbow           flank (side)　横腹
肘　窩
the inside of the elbow       waist　腰（腹まわりの最大部）
(the bend of the arm)
                              the small of the back　仙骨部
橈側　radial surface
(the inside of the wrist)     buttocks　尻（後部最大面積部）
尺側　ulnar surface
(the outside of the wrist)    hip　腰（尻まわりの最大部）
手の甲　the back of the hand
                              seat　尻（腰掛けに当たる部分）

        手の平　palm
                              thigh　もも
膝の曲がり皺
the crease of the knee        the back (hollow, bend) of the knee
膝のおさらの先端              膝窩部
the bottom of the knee cap
                              calf　ふくらはぎ
        すね　shin
                              the outside of the ankle
                              外側のくるぶし
        足の甲　instep
                              the inside of the ankle
        土ふまず　arch         内側のくるぶし

                              the sole of the foot　足の裏
        かかと　heel
```

Fig.7　Common names for parts of the body
　　　word phrases indicate radiographic landmarks（連語は撮影時の指標を表す）

Appendix 3
KEY EXPRESSIONS ON THE SPOT
その場での重要表現

1. At the registration counter　受付で
1）May I ask where you are from?　どこの国の方ですか（Which country 〜 ?）
2）Did someone recommend this clinic?　誰かの紹介者ですか（Who brought you here?）
　　cf. What brought you here?：どういたしましたか（i.e. What is the trouble?）
3）Where is the registration window for first visit?　初診窓口
4）Let me see your health insurance certificate and ID card.　保険証と診察券
5）Where is the admission / discharge window?　入退院窓口
6）Take this prescription to a pharmacy.　薬局に処方箋を持っていく
7）Could you itemize the fee for services?　診療の明細を教えていただけませんか
8）What are the clinical (office) hours?　診療時間
9）I'd like to come see a doctor late afternoon.　午前遅くに診察に行きたい
　　cf. I'll go to see him off at the airport.：見送りに行く
10）When is the last registration time for the morning?　午前の最終受け付け時間
11）I'd rather visit my father out of office hours.　勤務時間外に見舞いに行く
12）What are the visiting hours?　面会時間

2. Directions to patients　患者さんへの指示
On the examination table　検査台での体位
1）Hop up here on the table.　寝台に上がってください
2）Sit down on the table.　そこに座ってください
3）Lie on your back.（in the supine position）　仰向きに寝てください（仰臥位に）
4）Lie on your stomach.（in the prone position）　腹ばいに（腹臥位に）
5）Turn your face this way（or, the other way）．顔をこちらに
　　cf. Face this way.：体全体を
6）Turn over on your back again.　ぐるっと回ってまた仰向きに
7）Lie on your left side.（in the left recumbent position）
　　左を下にして（左側臥位）

8) Roll over onto your right side, this time. 　ごろりと右下になるまで回って
9) Turn halfway toward your left side.（in the RPO*¹ or LAO position）
左臥位の斜位
10) Place your legs out straight. 　足をまっすぐに伸ばして
11) Bend both knees and bring them together. 　両膝を曲げて，それを閉じる
12) I'm not getting fresh*². 　ごめんなさいね
13) You may sit up now. 　起き上がって（座って）ください
cf. Stand up：立ち上がる
14) Wait until I swing you up. 　起こしてあげますので待っていてください
15) Climb down from the table over here. 　ここから降りてください

＊1　臥位の場合は原則としてRPO（Right Posterior Oblique）を使用する。立位で用いるLAO（Left Anterior Oblique）と同じ斜位であるが，臥位でLAOを用いるときは，臥位でのLAOと明記する。

＊2　To get fresh with：（女性に対して）なれなれしいの意味。恥骨結合などを触るときにぜひ必要な表現。次のようにフォローする。
This part is the landmark for the x-ray.

3. Upright examination 　立位検査の体位

1) Move a little to your right. 　ちょっと右へ寄ってください
2) Take a half step to your left. 　半歩左へ
3) You're leaning to the right. 　右に傾いています
4) Relax your shoulders, please. 　肩の力を抜いてください
5) Don't bend over, keep your back straight and your head up 　かがまないで，背筋をまっすぐ伸ばして顔を正面にして
i.e. Don't flex but extend your back：屈曲でなく，伸展
6) Put your arms at your side. <or> Rest the palms of your hands against your thighs (i.e. neutral position). 　両手を脇に（中間位）
7) Turn your palms so they face out. <or> Put the back of your hands on your hips (i.e. supinate the arms). 　手のひらを外に向けて（回外位）
8) Drop your head forward and tuck your chin in. (i.e. flexion of neck)
下を向いて（首の屈曲）
9) Lift your chin as high as possible and let your head drop back. (i.e. hyperextension) 　できるだけ顎を上げて（過伸展）
10) Let me correct the position. 　位置を直します

11) Don't help me.　自分勝手に動かないで
12) Roll your shoulders forward and put your hands on your hips, palms up.
　　肩を前に回して手を腰に，手のひらは表にして
13) Clasp your hands behind your head and bring your elbows in（i.e. Adduct the elbows）.　　頭の後ろで手を組んで，肘を狭めてください（両肘の内転）

4. Expressions of breathing　呼吸

1) Take a deep breath.　大きく息を吸って
2) Breathe in and out repeatedly.　息を吸ったり吐いたりしてください
3) Stop breathing, please.　息を止めて
4) Hold your breath. Don't breathe.　そのまま息を止めていて
5) I need you to be still.　じっとして動かないで
6) You may breathe but try not to move.　息はしてもよいが，動かないように
7) OK. You can breathe now.　はい，息を吸ってもいいですよ
8) Let your stomach out（hold it in）.　お腹を膨らます（へこませる）
9) Hold on a minute. <or> Stay as you are.　そのままの姿勢でいてください

5. Preparation for dressing or undressing　更衣の準備

1) Pull the trousers up to your knee.　膝までまくり上げる
2) Roll up your sleeve to your elbow, please.　肘までまくる
3) Just undo the zipper（buttons）to show the chest.　チャック（ボタン）をはずす
4) Undress to the waist, please.　上半身裸になる
5) Take off everything from the waist up.　上半身裸になる
6) May I leave on my undershirt?　アンダーシャツを着ていてもいいか
7) Buttons or the like sometimes show on the x-rays.　ボタンやそのような物は写る
8) Strip to the waist, except for your bra.　ブラだけ残して上半身裸
9) Bras and underpants sometimes include metal or hard objects.　ブラやパンツには硬いものがついているときがある
10) You'll need another x-ray with additional radiation.　撮り直しで余分に被ばくする
11) After you get undressed, put this gown on.　脱ぎ終わったら，このガウンを着る
12) You'll need to take off your glasses.　眼鏡も外す
13) Put your belongings in the basket.　持ち物はかごの中へ
14) All finished. You may change into your clothes.　着替えてもよい
15) Don't rush. Take your time.　急がなくてもよい

6. Before and after an examination　検査の前後

1) How soon will it be before my turn?　私の順番はあと何番目
2) Your number will come up soon.　すぐ順番がくる
3) Please be seated. We'll call you soon.　お呼びしますので，座って待っていて
4) It's your turn. I'm sorry you had to wait so long.　順番ですよ，お待たせしました
5) The attendant will be outside.　付き添いの方は外でお待ちください
6) Follow me please.　こちらへどうぞ
7) Let's take a picture of your chest.　胸の写真を撮りましょう
8) Let's take a CT just in case.　念のためにCT検査をしましょう
9) Let's take an MRI for a thorough checkup.　精密検査のためにMRI検査を
10) Let's take an ultrasound to check movement of your heart.　超音波で心臓検査を
11) Let me apply gel so the ECG electrodes firmly stick to the skin.　心電計の電極がぴったりと皮膚につくようゼリーを塗る
12) Are you sure you are not expecting*1?　妊娠していないでしょうね
13) Do you know the 10-day rule*2 where you have less chance of pregnancy?　10日ルールを知っていますか。その間は妊娠の可能性が低いということを
14) Have you had a barium examination in the last week?　ここ1週間以内に胃の検査を
15) Please wait a few minutes while your bill is prepared.　伝票を用意しますので
16) Now, go to the second floor for blood and urine tests.　血液・尿検査
17) Oh, you're being paged for the clinical tests.　検査室で（マイクで）呼んでいますよ
18) Go pay at the third window on the first floor.　一階の3番窓口へ
19) Take care of yourself.　お大事に

　　*1　妊娠の婉曲表現
　　*2　The 10 days following the first menstruation, in which the possibility of a pregnancy is remote.

7. Nursing care　看護処置

1) Let me apply a cold compress to relieve the pain.　冷湿布
2) Apply the hot compress after the pain has gone.　温湿布は痛みがとれてから
3) I put some salve on it.　塗り薬をつけました
4) Put your hands out with your thumbs up.　親指を上にして手を置いて
5) Don't tense up. Try to let your body go limp.　緊張しないで，体の力を抜いて

6) Relax your arm and I'll clean it a bit with some alcohol.　アルコールで消毒する
7) Clench your fist firmly so the vein stands out.
　　血管が見えるように，こぶしをしっかり握って
8) It won't hurt too much, only a slight sting.
　　そんなに痛くない，ちくりとするだけ
9) Don't bend your arm or take off the tape until the bleeding stops.
　　血が止まるまで腕を曲げたりテープを剥がないで
10) Make a loose fist. I'll put this rubber tube（tourniquet）around your arm.
　　指の力を抜いて。ゴムチューブを腕に巻きます
11) Your blood pressure is 150 over 90, a little bit high for your age.
　　血圧は高い方が150で（systolic BP：収縮期血圧），低い方が90で（diastolic BP：拡張期血圧），年の割に高い
12) Spread your fingers. I'll apply a bandage around the thumb.
　　指をひろげて。親指に包帯を巻きます
13) Don't take off the dressing until the bleeding stops.
　　血が止まるまでガーゼをとらないで

8. Cold and pollen allergy　風邪と花粉症
1) I caught a bad cold.　風邪をひいた
2) I have a stuffy nose.　鼻づまり
3) I feel chilly.　寒気がする
4) I'm cold.（体が）寒い　*cf. He is coldhearted.*：（態度が）冷たい
5) I have a splitting headache.　頭ががんがんする
6) I have a smarting pain in the back of my head.　後頭部がずきずきする
7) My head is fuzzy.　頭がぼおっとする
8) Have you had a flu shot?　インフルエンザの予防注射を打っていますか
9) You seem to have a high fever.　高熱があるようですね
10) I feel feverish.　熱っぽく感じる
11) Can I take both the pain killer and medicine for fever together?　痛み止め（analgestic：鎮痛剤）と，熱さまし（antipyretic：解熱剤）を同時に飲む
12) I am suffering from a pollen allergy.　花粉症で悩んでいる
13) I have a runny nose.　鼻水が出る
14) My eyes are watering.　涙が出る
15) I had a sneezing bout.　連発でくしゃみが出る

9. Trauma and generative symptoms　外傷と退行性の症状

1) I got a strained back（lower back pain）　ぎっくり腰
2) I have a slipped disk.　椎間板ヘルニア　(i.e. herniation: ヘルニア形成)
3) I caught my fingers in the door.　ドアに指を挟んだ
4) I have shoulder stiffness.　肩こり
5) I have a frozen shoulder.　五十肩
6) I got a whiplash injury in a car accident.　むちうち症
7) I sprained my ankle.　足首をひねった（捻挫した）
8) I sprained my finger.　突き指をした
9) I sprained my neck while sleeping.　寝ちがい
10) I dislocated my left shoulder.　脱臼
11) I broke my leg.　脚を折った ＜or＞ I got a fracture in my leg.
12) I scraped my arm.　腕をすりむいた
13) My leg was bruised.　打撲傷を負った
14) My leg fell asleep（numb）.　しびれた
15) My leg got a cramp.　痙攣した
16) My leg had a torn muscle.　肉離れを起こした
17) I got a burn on my hand.　やけどをした

10. Patient's complaints and symptoms　患者の症状と愁訴

1) He has red specks on his face.　顔に虹斑がある　(i.e. erythema: 紅斑)
2) He has severe hives.　蕁麻疹がある　(i.e. urticaria: 蕁麻疹)
3) His heart is beating violently.　鼓動が激しい　(i.e. pulpitiations: 動悸)
4) His pulse is fast（low）.　(i.e. tachycardia: 頻脈)，(i.e. bradycardia: 遅脈)
5) He has an irregular pulse.　(i.e. arrhythmia: 不整脈)
6) He turned very pale.　真っ青になった。(i.e. cyanosis: チアノーゼ)
7) I have rapid（slow）breathing.　(i.e. tachypnea: 頻呼吸)，(i.e. bradypnea: 徐呼吸)
8) I feel a squeezing pain in my heart.　絞るような痛み　(i.e. angina: 狭心症)
9) I have difficulty in breathing.　息苦しい　(i.e. dyspnea: 呼吸困難)
10) I get short of breath.　息切れ　(i.e. shallow breathing: 表在呼吸)
11) I feel like throwing up（vomiting）.　吐き気　(i.e. nausea: 悪心)
12) I feel dizzy spells when I stand up.　立ち眩みがする
13) I'm anemic.　貧血気味　(i.e. anemia: 貧血)

14) I feel light-headed　ふらつく
15) He passed out（fainted）．気絶した

11. Expressions of pain　痛みの表現
1) Pain radiates to the tip of my toe.　痛みが足先まで放散する
2) Pain comes and goes in regular intervals.　周期的にやってくる
3) The injury throbs.　傷がズキンズキンする
4) The injury stings.　傷がチクチクする
5) The injury burns.　傷がヒリヒリする
6) The injury is so painful that I can't sleep.　痛むが激しくて寝られない
7) My stomach has a dull pain.　胃に鈍い痛みがある
8) My stomach has a sharp pain.　鋭い痛みがある
9) My stomach has a gripping pain.　胃がシクシク痛む
10) My stomach has a strange pain.　胃に不気味な痛みがある
11) My stomach has a biting pain.　胃に刺すような痛みがある
12) My stomach has a tingling pain.　胃がキリキリ痛む
13) The pain was relieved (eased).　痛みが和らいだ
14) The pain is lighter than ever.　いつもよりいくらかは和らいでいる

Appendix 4
THE CONSTRUCTION OF ENGLISH
構文別英会話集

1. Causative verbs　使役動詞
1) I **made** him drive my car.　命令または強要
2) I **let** him drive my car.　許可
3) She **made** me **let** him drive my car.
　（酔っているので）彼に運転させろと強いた
4) I **got** him **to** drive my car.　巧みに～させる
5) I **had** him drive my car.　依頼
6) I'll **have** to have my car **driven** by him.　目的語が物のときは過去分詞

　　(1) We **made** him **feel** at ease.　安心させた
　　(2) We **had** him **relax**.　リラックスさせた
　　(3) Help the patient rise by **having** him **put** his hands on your shoulders.
　　　　患者さんが立ち上がるときに肩を貸してあげなさい。
　　(4) Have you **had** any x-rays **taken** of your stomach recently?
　　　　最近胃のX線写真を撮ったことがありますか。

2. Subjunctive mood　仮定法
1) If you **studied** hard you would pass the exam.　現状の反対を仮定
2) If I **had studied** hard I might have passed the exam.　過去に関する遺憾の意
3) Even a pig **would** climb a tree **if** you flatter him enough.　ありそうもないない未来
4) **Would** you mind my smoking here?　丁寧な依頼

　　(1) Consider how you **would like to be** treated if you **were** a patient.
　　　　もしあなたが患者だったら
　　(2) He **would have been** more cooperative if you **had told** him what was going to be done to him.
　　(3) Treat patients with the same concern that you **would** appreciate if you **were** ill.　あなたが病気であったとき，ありがたいと思う気配り

(4) When a delay occurred, I **should've given** them an update and explanation as to the schedule change.　待ち時間が延びたとき，そのつど（患者さんに）情報を伝えるべきだった。

3. Inanimate subject　物主構文

1) **What** made her so sad?　どうしてそんなに悲しかったのだろう
2) **One thing** led to another.　次々と事が起こった
3) **Business** took me there.　仕事でそこに行った
4) **The year 1986** saw the tragic space shuttle Challenger accident.
5) **The news** says that the cause of the accident is not yet clear.

(1) **Experience** has taught us that it is completely safe.
　　経験から安全とわかっている
(2) **This evaluation** might lead to an erroneous conclusion.
　　誤った結果を生じるだろう
(3) **Compromise** often emerges out of the conflict of argument.
　　意見の衝突から妥協が
(4) **This equipment** frees us from the time-consuming need to have the patient lie on the table.　手間のかかる〜をしないですむ

4. Comparison　比較

1) She pretended to be ten years younger **than** she **really was**.　10歳さばを読む
2) He is not **as** smart **as** his wife.　i.e. His wife is smarter than he is.
3) I am older **than he thinks** I am.　彼が思っているより老けている

(1) Tokyo is 1.5 **times as** expensive **as** any other city in the world in commodity prices.　東京の市場物価はどの世界の都市に比べて1.5倍高い
　　c.f. Tokyo is expensive.
(2) **Nowhere else** in the world **is there** a more expensive city than Tokyo.
　　世界中のどこに東京より物価の高い都市があるだろうか。
(3) Any other city is less expensive than Tokyo **by 20 percent or more**.
　　20パーセント以上安い
(4) A smoker's mortality due to lung cancer is **as much as** 53 times higher **than** that of a non-smoker.　喫煙者の肺癌による死亡率は非喫煙者に比べ53倍

も高い（強調表現）
(5) It is easier **for a camel to** go through the eye of a needle than **for a rich man to** enter into the kingdom of God.（Matthew 19:24）
金持ちが神の国に入るよりは，ラクダが針の穴を通るほうが，ずっとやさしい。（マタイ19:24）＜誇張した比較で **much** easier を言外に含む＞

5. Insertion and ellipsis　挿入と省略
1) What **do you think** he is?　彼の職業は何だと思いますか。
2) Today, **according to the newspaper,** about one third of the power supply comes from nuclear energy.
今日，新聞によると，日本の電力の1/3は原子力に負う
3) The two modalities, **PTC and ERCP**, are not alternatives but complements to each other.　経皮経肝性胆管造影と内視鏡的膵・胆管造影は互いに競合でなく補完し合う
4) The theory **the doctor said** he first advocated has been widely accepted worldwide.
自分が最初に提唱したと言っているその理論（本当かどうかはわからない）
5) How soon **do you think** CT will completely take the place of invasive angiography?
CTが観血的な血管造影に完全に取って代わるのはどのくらい先
6) Correct the errors. **If any**, there would be very few.
あったにしても，ごくまれだろう
7) **If need be**, this can be manually interrupted to space the scan more closely together.
必要なら手動で，もう少し密に（超音波の）スキャンができる

6. Adverbial phrases　副詞句
1) now that/ in that / providing that
　～からには／～の意味において／もし～ならば
2) so that / once（that）/ given that　～のため／～からには／～の場合は
3) no matter how / no more than　どんなに～しても／たかだか
4) the more ～ / the more ～　～すればするほど／～になる
5) When it comes to / which ever　～のこととなると／どちらか

　　(1) I've got to take it easy **now that** my doctor has told me clearly that my case is benign.　はっきり良性と言われたので気が楽になった

(2) Empathy differs from actions following compassion or sympathy **in that** empathetic actions rise above one's logic.
Empathy は理性を超えた感情であるという意味において

(3) The care provided will be more effective **given that** more sophisticated equipment is used. 高度な装置が使用されれば
cf. **Given** the problem **that** we experienced with the conventional technique we decided to try a new technique.：過去の経験で〜に問題があるのを知っていたので

(4) **When it comes to** deliver**ing** radiation to a tumor containing volume with minimum irradiation, brachytherapy is **second to none**.
最小限の線量で，病巣部容積を照射することにかけては，密封小線源治療に並ぶものはない

(5) When you cannot decide, chose **whichever** is least.
迷うなら，どちらか少ない方を

(6) She would have succeeded in loosing weight, **provided that** she complied with the diet regimen. ダイエット食事療法を守っていた**なら**／（〜したろうに） cf. provided that：〜なら（〜する）；条件付きで（on condition that ~）Appendix 5, 62）参照

7. Inversions　倒置構文

1) **Little did** I dream I'd ever see you again.
また会えるなんて，夢にも思わなかった
2) **Such was** the story he confided in me.　彼が打ち明けたのは，そんな話だった
3) **Incredible it** is that he's kept single so far.　まだ独身だなんて，信じられない

　(1) This is the clinical ID card on which **can be written** the patient's name, age, sex and other information.
氏名，年齢，性別　その他の情報が書かれた診察券

　(2) **Nowhere else** in medical imaging **is there** more dependency on the skill of the equipment operator than in ultrasound scanning.
超音波ほど操作者の腕次第の画像技術はない

　(3) **Included are** many that test non-hormonal peptides, drugs, enzymes and so on.　この検査は，非ペプチドホルモン〜を含む（倒置構文で頭でっかちを防ぐ）

Appendix 5
100 SELECTED IDIOMATIC EXPRESSIONS
慣用表現100選

1. **Aside from**[1] your hospital, I would like to see **what** the American medical system is really **all about**[2].
   あなたの病院だけでなく，アメリカの医療制度の**本質**もみたい。
2. I'll **see to it that** you can get to me at once.
   すぐに私に会えるように**おはからい**します。
3. Your remark isn't **relevant to**[3] the point we're discussing.
   あなたの発言は今の問題に**直接関係**ありません。
4. We're still **at opposite poles**, but we'll **leave it at that**.
   まだ意見に**大きな差**がありますが，そこまでにしておきましょう。
5. You must try to **meet us half way** or this discussion won't go anywhere.
   お互いに**歩み寄らない**とどうにもまとまりません。
6. He is **getting carried away with** his own research, and not concentrating on the group work.
   彼は個人研究に**図に乗って**，協同作業には関心がない。
7. Don't **go out of your way** on my account. Don't try to be so polite.
   私のために**わざわざそう（する）**しないでください。
8. **For the time being**, let's just wait and see.
   当分は様子をみることにしましょう。
9. Our department has **beefed up** the staff and has let them **take up different assignments**.
   わが部署では職員を**補強**し，それぞれの仕事に**専念**させている。
10. We can't expect even **a fraction of** success if the staff doesn't really **get down to**[4] work on it.
    本腰を入れ（る）ないとわずかな成功も望めない。

---

1) ～aside, ～は別として
2) ex. That is what it's all about. それに尽きる
3) or, associated with
4) or, take a serious attitude to

11. Turn it **the other way around**, not clockwise, but counter clockwise.
    逆に回しなさい，右じゃなくて左側に。
12. The magazine **holds up to**[5] 100 sheets of film.
    このマガジンはフィルム100枚まで**収容**できます。
13. The doctor **speaks highly of** this equipment.
    この装置は医師の**評判**がよい。
14. There is **a wide spectrum of** opinion regarding that machine.
    この装置の評判は**まちまち**だ。
15. **Given a choice**, you need to **go over**[6] both of the specifications before deciding.
    どちらか選ぶとなると両方の仕様を**丹念に調べ**（る）なければならない。
16. **Suffice it to say that** this machine should only be used by the operator **best equipped to** handle it.
    熟練者のみが操作すべきであるというにとどめておきましょう。
17. You are **way ahead of** us in this technique. **For the life of me**, I can't see how we can **rank up with** you.
    あなたの技術は**はるかに進んで**います。どうみても追いつくのは無理のようです。
18. The statement "Better safe than sorry" is **never more true than when** applied to radiation safety.
    "安全第一主義"ということが放射線の安全で**特に痛感される**。
19. **Developing good rapport** with your patients will **give rise to** more cooperation on their part.
    患者との**信頼関係**が増すともっと患者の協力が得られるようになる。
20. You have to **live up to**[7] the confidence your patients place in you.
    患者の信頼に**応え**（る）なければなりません。
21. You must **keep an eye on** the children all the time that you are treating them.
    子供から**目を離さない**よう。
22. You should try to **prepare** children **for** an examination instead of **tricking** them **into** it.
    だまして検査を受けさせるより，なだめてその気に（覚悟）させることだ。
23. If you show a little bit of kindness to the child, he **is bound to** like you.

---

5) cf. stands up to〜　〜まで耐える
6) or, go through cf. skin, run（over, through）　ざっと調べる
7) or, meet, fulfill

少しでも親切にすると，きっと子供はあなたを好き**になる**。

24. The doctor finally **broke the news** to the patient that his illness was serious.
医者はついに患者の病気の重いことを**打ち明けた**。

25. Don't try to **cheer** the patient **up by** divulg**ing** all that you know about his illness.
病状を知らせて患者を**元気づける**のはやめなさい。

26. **It may very well be that** he won't want to be treated as such an old patient.
たぶん年寄り扱いをされたくないの**かもしれない**。

27. Don't **make light of** the children's complaints, but **make the most of** them so that you can understand them better.
子供を理解するため，訴えを**軽くみ（る）**ないでできるだけ**重視（する）**しなさい。

28. It's surprising that the system **comes to be that** expensive.
それが**そんなに**高いとは驚きだ。

29. Just because it's easy to handle, **it doesn't follow that** it doesn't require expertise.
操作が簡単だからといっても，専門知識がいらない**ということでない**。

30. Cholesterol or lipid cannot **get along with** water.　なじまない

31. LDL also plays an important role **as such**, bringing cholesterol to the organs.
LDL は**それなり**の役割を果たしている。

32. Cytokine and vitamin D **go hand in hand** to keep healthy bones.
サイトカインとビタミンDは骨を健康に保つ**相乗作用がある**。

33. This is **referred to as** a Geiger-Mueller counter, and it's **named after** the inventors.
発明者の**名にちなんで**ガイガー・ミュラーカウンタ**と呼ばれている**。

34. The image is reasonable, **not to say** beautiful.
美しいとまでは**いえないまでも**まあまあだ。

35. "Micro-calcifications" they said, and looked at me **as if to say**"nonsense".
「微小石灰化」と彼らは言って，馬鹿な**といわんばかりに**私を見た。

36. **It was not until** the advent of the electronic scanner that they began to **think much of** it.
大したものだと思い始めたのは電子スキャナが出現してからのことであった。

37. Its success is **owed in part to** the efforts of pioneers **and in part to** the development of electronics.
その成功は先駆者の努力と電子技術の発達に**負う**。

38. The images in the early days were extremely ambiguous, **so much that** they looked

just like a gathering of clouds.
当初の画像はまったく不鮮鋭**もいいとこ**，まるで雲のかたまりを見ているようだった。

39. By integrated diagnosis, we never mean that you should adopt just **any** modality **that comes in handy**.
    総合画像診断とは，**手当たり次第に**撮影方式を採用することではない。

40. The gold standard means the criterion on which we **finally fall back**.
    gold standard とは**最後に頼れる**診断基準である。

41. The patient **might as well** be sent for dynamic CT immediately after angiography, since the catheter is already in place.
    すでにカテーテルが入っているのだから，**どうせなら**アンギオの直後にCTを**したほうがよい**。

42. Positron images are not yet satisfactory. **If anything**, they **fall short of our expectations**.
    ポジトロン画像はまだ満足ではない。**どちらかといえば期待外れ**だ。

43. The coagulation **holds up**[8] the agent passing through the precapillaries.
    凝固により薬が前毛細管を通るのを**阻止する**。

44. A machine that costs a lot of money to keep up will prove more expensive **in the long run**.
    維持費の多くかかる機械は**長い目でみれば**高くつく。

45. The initial cost of such expensive equipment cannot **be written off**.
    そんなに高い購入価格では**減価償却**できない。

46. Without the A-C bypass operation, most of the patients who **come down with** ischemic heart disease **would otherwise be** dead.
    A-Cバイパス手術がなかったら，多くの虚血性心疾患に**冒された**患者は助か**らないだろう**。

47. You can see the four chambers head-on **by virtue of** the angle view.
    アングルビューの**おかげで**四室を正面に見ることができる。

48. **Rather than** just sit and wait for death, the patient **might as well** undergo the operation.
    座して死を待つよりは手術を受けた**ほうがました**。

49. I am sorry to say that only a few patients, **if any**, will survive the disease.
    残念ながらその病気で助かる患者は，**あったにせよ**，ごくまれだ。

---

8) ex. hold up the line　（人の）流れを阻む

50. **Given** the size of the superconductive magnet, you better be prepared to provide ample space **so as to** accommodate the MRI scanner.
    超電導磁石の大きさを気にする**ならば**，MRI装置を収容する**ために**広い場所を用意したほうがよい。

51. That **accounts for quite a small**[9] portion of total heart disease.
    それは心疾患全体のうちで**非常に大きな割合を占める**。

52. Thereafter, we leave the calculation to the planning system to do in **its own way**.
    その後の計算は治療計画システムの**なすがままにまかせる**。

53. Kidney damage is a product of the disease **by and large**.
    腎障害は**大体**において通風の結果である

54. Unless you **give** it **full play** in practice, it will turn out to be **good for nothing**.
    実際に**実力を発揮**（する）できなければ，**無用の長物**となる。

55. As a matter of fact, the regulations **put into effect** in those days **conflict with** the actual situation today.
    実のところ，あの頃に**施行された**法規は現在の実情に**合わない**。

56. **It goes without saying that** anything that can be done by that method can be done just as well by this one.
    あの方法でできるものならば，これらの方法でも同様にできる**のはいうまでもない**。

57. **When it comes to** figuring out plans, he is **second to none**.
    計画を考え出すことにかけては，彼に**並ぶものはない**。

58. It wasn't his idea, per se, but he **had** a lot **to do with** it.
    彼自身のアイデアではなかったが，**かかわり合いは大いにある**。

59. The medical use of radium **dates back to** the time of Madame Curie.
    ラジウムの医学への応用は，キュリー夫人の時代に**さかのぼる**。

60. We considered using cesium instead of the radium, but **thought better of**[10] it.
    ラジウムの代わりにセシウムを使うことを考えたが**考え直してやめた**。

61. It may **stand to reason** that many Japanese are sensitive to anything related to nuclear energy.
    日本人がいかなる核エネルギーにも敏感なのは**当然だ**。

62. **Now that** all the test tools have been prepared, the Q. A. program will succeed **provided that** the staff is determined to **bring it off**.

---

9) cf. quite a few　たくさんの

10) or, had second thoughts about

道具がすべて揃った**からには**，皆が**やり通す**決意がある**ならば**このQAプログラムは成功する。

63. The program didn't work out **inasmuch as** the Q. C. leader couldn't get along with the **rank and file** members.
    このQAプログラムは，指導者が**部下**とうまくいかなかった**ので**成功していない。

64. They **came to their wits end** when trying to decide who should pay for the new equipment if it were damaged during testing.
    テストの最中に機械が故障したら誰が補償するのかで，**はたと途方**にくれた。

65. Quality assurance has a wider connotation than just that of quality control **in that** it includes quality administration procedures as well.
    品質保証は行政的管理も含む**という点で**，品質管理よりは意味が広い。

66. Q.C. programs start with **breaking down** the statistics and then trying to **figure out** which counter measures should be taken.
    QCプログラムは統計を**分析する**ことから始まり，次に対策を**考え出す**。

67. This microdensitometer **renders** operator's intervention **unnecessary in terms of** data analysis.
    このマイクロデンシトメータは，データ分析に関しては操作者の介入を**不要にする**。

68. Is that why you just **looked over**[11] the equipment performance specifications and didn't **go through** them carefully?
    装置の仕様を，ただ目を通しただけで丹念に調べ（る）なかったせいじゃないの。

69. When we develop film manually, a small variation in exposure can be compensated for by "**cooking**" the development process.
    手現像のときは少しぐらいの濃度変化は現像で**手加減**できた。

70. Microprocessors are gradually **finding their way** into controlling all functions of x-ray exposure.
    マイクロプロセッサーがだんだんに曝射制御のすべての面に**入りつつある**。

71. Human error **makes up** three quarters of the retakes. Machine problems constitute the rest.

---

11) cf. look through 〜を十分調べる

操作ミスが撮り直しの3/4を**占める**。残りは装置の故障である。

72. **The thing is**[12], nobody **straightened up** the room after the test.
    要は，テストの後に誰も部屋を**片づけ（る）**なかったことだ。

73. We'll talk about the next step of the process once you've **straightened out** the problems in the first step.
    最初の問題を**片づけて**から次の段階について話し合いましょう。

74. We gave a liberal estimation of possible damages, to be **on the safe side**.
    大事をとって，被害を過大評価した。

75. I want you to recognize the result **as such**, whatever that may be.
    結果がどうであれ，**それなりに**評価してもらいたい。

76. Cost and machine downtime are by and large **inversely related**; that is, the more you invest in the program, the less likely the machine is to break down.
    投資と機械の非稼動時間は，大体において**相反関係にある**。すなわち，投資するほど故障は減るものだ。

77. Try it. Now is the time to **show your stuff**.
    やってみなさい。今こそ**腕の見せ所**だ。

78. If we could have such a specialist, **so much the better**.
    専門家がいれば**それに超したことはない**。

79. You should have a job you feel worth living for, **if you do at all**, work which motivates your morale.
    どうせなら，生きがいのある職業を選ぶべきだ，やる気を起こさせるような。

80. **Spare me the details**, just give me the bottom line.
    細かいことは**抜きにして**，結論だけを言ってくれ。

---

12) or, the point is,　（注）is の後のコンマはなくてもよい。

Appendix 6
COFFEE BREAK VOCABULARY
歓談用語句集

Education：教育

教育問題	educational issue
生涯教育	lifelong education
卒後教育	post-graduate education
国立（官立）学校	national（or government）school
私立学校	private school
都立（市立）学校	metropolitan（or municipal）school
義務教育	compulsory education
教育年限	terms of education
職業教育	vocational education
専門学校	specialty school
短期大学	junior college
四年制（単科）大学	four-year college
教養科目	liberal arts
専門課程	professional course
臨床実習	clinical practice
学部	faculty or department
選択科目	elective subject
必須科目	required subject
単位制度	point（or credit）system
授業料	school fee or tuition
試験科目	subject of examination
検定試験	certificate examination
資格試験	qualification examination
国家試験	governmental or state examination
学士号	bachelor's degree or baccalaureate
修士号	master's degree
博士号	doctoral degree

大学生	undergraduate
大学院生	graduate student
同窓生	alumnus（pl. alumni）
二学期制	semester system
三学期制	trimester system
四学期制	quarter system
受験地獄	examination hell
教育ママ	education mama
予備校	cram school
有名校	famous school
少年犯罪	juvenile delinquency
いじめ	（school）bullying

Social standing：社会的地位

身分法	status law
履歴	curriculum vitae or personal history
国籍	nationality
婚姻（未婚，既婚）	marital status（single, married）
自宅（会社）住所	home（business）address
免許	license
会員資格	professional membership
任用	appointment
賃金	allowances
初任給	starting salary（pay）
本俸	regular salary
名目賃金	nominal salary
手取り給料	take-home pay
昇給	increase in pay（salary）
年功加俸	longevity pay
能率給	efficiency pay
超過勤務手当	overtime pay
給与改善	betterment of salary
週五日制	five-day work week

有給休暇	paid holiday
夏期賞与	mid-summer bonus
年末賞与	year-end bonus
特別給与	fringe benefit
職務手当	service allowance
家族手当	family allowance
調整手当	adjustment allowance
食事手当	lunch allowance
危険手当	danger money（hazard pay）
住宅手当	housing allowance
控除	deduction
雇用保険	unemployment insurance
所得税	earned income tax
住民税	resident tax
厚生年金	welfare annuity
退職金	retirement compensation
恩給	pension

Medical system：医療制度

老人保険法	Health Care Act for the Aged
成人病検診	adults' disease checkup
成人病（老人病）	geriatric diseases
生活習慣病	lifestyle disease
寝たきり老人	bed-ridden old person
ボケ老人	feeble-minded old person
老人性痴呆症	senile dementia
福祉行政	welfare administration
診療報酬	diagnostic rewards
医療給付	medical benefit
加算制度	sliding scale system
重度身体障害者	seriously disabled patient
健康手帖	health notebook
集団検診	mass screening

早期発見	early detection
生命保険	life insurance
毎月の掛金	monthly installment
保険料	premium
カルテ	clinical chart
指示標	indication slips
照射録	exposure report
検査報告	examination report
会計報告	accounting report
診察券	consultation ticket or ID card
急救患者	first-aid patient
車椅子患者	wheelchair patient
担架患者	litter patient
寝台患者	stretcher patient
松葉杖患者	patient on crutches
入院（外来）患者	in（out）patient
外来	out-patient clinic
入退院センター	admissions department
医療技術者	co-medicals
臨床検査技師（学士号）	medical technologist
臨床検査技師	medical laboratory technician
管理栄養士	dietitian
栄養士	dietetic technician
歯科衛生士	dental hygienist
歯科技工士	dental laboratory technician
理学療法士	physical therapist
作業療法士	occupational therapist
看護師	registered nurse
准看護師	practical nurse
開業看護師（大学院レベル）	nurse practitioner
助産師	nurse-midwife
保健師	public health nurse
医療物理士（総称）	medical physicist
放射線物理士（治療）	radiation physicist

薬剤師	pharmacist
薬局	dispensary
国立病院	national hospital
市民病院	municipal hospital
私立病院	private hospital
専門病院	special hospital
特殊病院	special hospital（authorized by law）
特殊承認医療機関	speciality authorized health insurance medical facility
特殊機能機関	special functinoing hospital
外科医	surgeon
外科病棟	surgical ward
内科医	physician
内科病棟	medical ward
婦人科医	gynecologist
産科医	obstetrician
整形外科医	orthopedic surgeon
小児科医	pediatrician
老人医学専門医	geriatrician
精神科医	psychiatrist
麻酔科医	anesthesiologist（専門）
麻酔士	anesthetist（代行）
頭頸外科医	head and neck surgeon
耳鼻咽喉科医	E.N.T. specialist（ear, nose, and throat）, or otorhinolaryngologist
眼科医	ophthalmologist
放射線医	radiologist
神経科医	neurologist
泌尿器科医	urologist
皮膚科医	dermatologist
歯科医	dentist
病理学者	pathologist
組織学者	histologist
細胞学者	cytologist
院長	the director（of a hospital）

所長	the head （of a center） or superintendent
部長	a director （of a department）
医長	a head （of a dept.）
管理者	superintendent
技師長	chief technologist
主任技師（無任所）	assistant chief technologist
主任技師（課長）	section chief technologist

General society：一般社会

高齢化社会	society of advanced age
学歴社会	academic career society
情報化社会	information-oriented society
技術革新	technological innovation
省力化	labor-saving efforts
行政改革	reform of administrative structure
行政指導	administrative guidance
行政処分	administrative measure
公正取引委員会	Fair Trade Commission commodity prices
物価	commodity prices
公共料金	public utilities charges
経済成長率	rate of economic growth
国民総生産	gross national product
貿易摩擦	trade friction
人事院	the National Personnel Authority
厚生労働省	the Ministry of Health, Labor and Welfare
文部科学省	the Ministry of Education, Culture, Sports, Science and Technology
経済産業省	the Ministry of Economy, Trade and Industry
外務省	the Ministry of Foreign Affairs
財務省	the Ministry of Finance
現大臣	present minister
前大臣	former minister
国家公務員	national public official （servant）

地方公務員	local public official (servant)
年功序列	promotion on seniority
成果主義	promotion on merits (merit system)
終身雇用制度	lifetime employment system
タテ社会	mental verticality or vertical society
根まわし	behind-the-scenes negotiation
腹芸	non-verbal communication
りん議制度	consensus-roll system
意思決定過程	decision-making process
停年制	age-limit system
温情主義	paternalism
閉鎖社会	close-knit society
本音と建前	words and actual intention

Structure of organization and academic meeting：組織の構造と学会

学際団体	multidisciplinary organization
職能団体	professional organization
社団法人	a corporation
財団法人	a foundation
特殊法人	government-affiliateted corporate
総会（および研究発表会）	the general assembly（and scientific meeting）
総会	the general meeting of the association
会長	chairman
副会長	vice-chairman
常務理事	managing director
代議員	representative or delegates
執行委員	executive committee
理事会	a board of directors （trustees）
評議会	council
技術委員会	technical committee
小委員会（分科会）	subcommittee
臨時委員会	ad hoc committee
常任委員会	standing committee

特別委員会	special committee
諮問委員会	advisory committee
準備委員会	preparatory committee
組織委員会	organizing committee
運営委員会	steering committee
作業班	working group
役員	executive committee member
本会議	plenary session
大会（大）	convention
会議（中）	congress
会議（小）	conference
正会員	regular member
準会員	associate member
随伴会員	social member
賛助会員	patronage member
名誉会員	honorary member
発表者	participant
登録者	registrant
登録用紙	registration form
登録費	registration fee
事務局	secretariat
事務職員	clerical staff
会費	membership fee
入会金	initiation fee
組織率	organization rate
会誌（機関誌）	journal（house organ）
学術プログラム	scientific program
教育展示	scientific exhibit
機器展示	technical exhibit
補習コース	refresher course
日本医師会	Japan Medical Association
日本歯科医師会	Japan Dental Association
日本看護協会	Japanese Nursing Association
日本放射線技師会	The Japan Association of Radiological Technologists

	（JART）
日本薬剤師会	Japan Pharmaceutical Association
日本臨床衛生検査技師会	Japanese Association of Medical Technologists
日本医学学術集会振興協会	Japan Federation of Medical Congress Promotion（JMCP）
日本医学放射線学会	Japan Radiological Society
日本放射線技術学会	Japanese Society of Radiological Technology（JSRT）
日本医学物理学会	The Japanese Association of Medical Physics
日本臨床工学技士会	Japan Association for Clinical Engineering Technologists
国際放射線技師会	International Society of Radiographers and Radiological Technicians（ISRRT）
米国医学物理学者協会	The American Association of Physicists in Medicine（AAPM）
国際放射線医学会議	International Congress of Radiology（ICR）
北米放射線学会	The Radiological Society of North America（RSNA）
国際協力機構	Japan International Cooperation Agency（JICA）

著者略歴

Marshall Smith　　保健科学博士，M.I.M.（国際経営学修士）
　1987年6月　　米国国際経営学大学院で M.I.M. 取得
　1988～1995年　大王製紙株式会社勤務（社長室秘書課）
　1995～1998年　東京大学大学院医学系研究科国際保健学専攻研究生
　1998年4月～　東京都立保健科学大学　客員助教授（保健，医学英語，および科学論文記述コース）
　2001年3月　　東京大学大学院医学系研究科博士課程国際保健学専攻卒業
　　　　　　　　Doctor of Health Science（保健科学博士）取得
　2001年4月～　帯広畜産大学助教授　現在に至る
　著　　書　　Tobacco: The Growing Epidemic (co-author). Springer-Verlag London Limited, 2000.
　　　　　　　Smith M., Iida Y.：看護・カルテ用語辞典．ナツメ社，2001．

佐藤　伸雄　　診療放射線技師（RT）
　1960年3月　　千葉大学附属診療エックス線技師学校卒業
　1960～1993年　癌研究会附属病院放射線診断科勤務
　1993～1997年　ウィスコンシン大学附属病院放射線技師学校非常勤講師
　1998年～　　北里大学医療衛生学部非常勤講師
　著　　書　　救急放射線診断マニュアル（監訳）．WHO/丸善，1988．
　　　　　　　放射線科における実践英会話（第2版）．医療科学社，1990．
　　　　　　　Encyclopedia of Radiographic Positioning (co-author). W.B. Saunders Company, 1993
　　　　　　　医療スタッフのための米会話（第2版）．医療科学社，2002．
　　　　　　　その他・技術専門書

|必携|

病院における実践英会話
医療従事者のための基本英語

価格はカバーに
表示してあります

2003年11月1日　第一版第1刷発行
2007年2月2日　第一版第2刷発行

著　者　Marshall Smith, 佐藤　伸雄Ⓒ
発行人　古屋敷　信一
発行所　株式会社 医療科学社
　　　　〒113-0033　東京都文京区本郷 3-23-1
　　　　TEL 03(3818)9821　FAX 03(3818)9371
　　　　ホームページ　http://www.iryokagaku.co.jp
　　　　郵便振替　00170-7-656570

ISBN978-4-86003-322-4　　　　（乱丁・落丁はお取り替えいたします）

本書の複製権・翻訳権・上映権・譲渡権・公衆送信権（送信可能化権を含む）は（株）医療科学社が保有します。

JCLS 〈（株）日本著作出版権管理システム委託出版物〉
本書の無断複写は著作権法上での例外を除き，禁じられています。
複写される場合は，そのつど事前に（株）日本著作出版権管理システム
（電話 03-3817-5670，FAX 03-3815-8199）の許諾を得てください。

医療スタッフのための米会話

著者：佐藤 伸雄　　校閲：Hunter M. Brumfield

- 本書は，従来みられなかった臨床医学に従事する人々のための英会話読本である。
- 放射線技術，看護，臨床検査技術に役立つ文型練習，医療現場での対話集，機器関連医療の専門英語を紹介している。
- 英文パターンの繰り返し練習を中心，基礎技術を題材にしたチャートに基づく文型練習，外国人来訪者（患者を含む）との対話，高度専門技術の知識・用語の把握，にて構成。

主要目次

Chapter 1. pattern Practice for Fundamental Expertises　基本技術のための文型練習
- Lesson 1　Basic Radiologic Technology　基本放射線技術
- Lesson 2　Nursing Techniques　看護技術
- Lesson 3　Medical Laboratory Technology　臨床検査技術
- Lesson 4　Job Description　職種紹介

Chapter 2. Typical Dialogues at Medical Sites　医療現場での対話集
- Lesson 5　Interaction with Patients　患者接遇
- Lesson 6　Interaction with Foreign Visitors　外国人客の接待
- Lesson 7　Comparison of Medical Systems　医療制度の比較

Chapter 3. Machine-Related Medical Techniques　機器関連医療技術
- Lesson 8　Computer-related Machinery　コンピュータ関連機器
- Lesson 9　Safety　安全
- Lesson 10　Diagnostic Tests and Procedures　診断検査・技術
- Lesson 11　Stete of the Art Medical Equipment　高度医療機器と先端技術

Supplement：Radio Exercise　ラジオ体操…体動表現

◆ B5判198頁　◆ 定価（本体 3,690 円＋税）　◆ ISBN 978-4-900770-27-0

画像診断機器工学 Q&A

編・著：佐藤 伸雄
著者：西山　篤・川村　守・小川　互・櫛谷 征昭

習っても，読んでも，聞いても，疑問が残るという方に，画像診断機器の理解に必要な原理論から応用まで，豊富な図解で説明。

主要目次

- I. 電源設備
- II. X線撮影・透視装置
  - X線源装置
  - 単相・三相装置
  - コンデンサ装置
  - インバータ装置
- III. 映像・画像診断装置
  - 映像装置
  - デジタル画像装置
  - 眼底写真装置
- IV. X線CT装置
  - CTの画像再構成法
- 画像評価と
  アーチファクト
- V. MR装置
  - NMR現象と
    パルスシーケンス
  - MR画像と
    アーチファクト
  - MR装置の構造
  - 高速GRE (gradient echo)
- と三次元画像表示法
- VI. 超音波画像装置
- 付録
  - 変圧器の原理
  - 共振回路の原理と応用
  - 機器工学のための自動制御
  - 指数関数と複素数
  - CTの画像再構成

◆ B5判210頁　◆ 定価（本体 3,800 円＋税）
◆ ISBN 978-4-900770-96-6

医療科学社　〒113-0033 東京都文京区本郷 3-23-1　TEL 03-3818-9821　FAX 03-3818-9371
http://www.iryokagaku.co.jp　（くわしくはホームページをご覧ください）

核災害に対する放射線防護
― 実践放射線防護学入門 ―

著者：高田 純

国民保護基本指針が想定する「核攻撃等または武力攻撃原子力災害」への対処措置として，地域の被曝医療体制への連帯のために，各都道府県の国民保護計画に関わる放射線安全担当者や防災担当者，さらに医療担当者に必須の基本知識。放射線被曝によるダメージ軽減のための核ハザード理論を明解・平易に提示する。

主要目次

- 核放射線の平和利用と放射線防護学
- 核災害事例の検証
- 線量の6段階区分
- 広島での空中核爆発と初期核放射線
- 空中核爆発時のグラウンド・ゼロでの現象
- 近距離生存者の線量回避
- 堅牢なコンクリート建造物内部の安全性
- 野村栄三さんの場合
- 核兵器攻撃時の対処法
- 空中核爆発後の核ハザードの減衰
- 原子力災害
- 原子力発電所事故災害の放射線影響
- 甲状腺の放射線防護と昆布
- 21世紀の脅威 ―戦術核兵器
- 核兵器テロと核ミサイル
- 核爆発と放射線防護
- 国民保護の現状／他

◆ A5判 84頁 ◆ 定価（本体 1,000円＋税）
◆ ISBN 978-4-86003-336-1

緊急被ばく医療テキスト

監修：青木 芳朗／前川 和彦

緊急被ばく医療おける診断と治療の実際を，核テロに対応した医療をも視野に入れて解説。加えて，生物・物理学的，および法律・制度的な基礎知識を整理して呈示し，原子力災害への医療体制のあり方を総括。

主要目次

序　論　緊急被ばく医療とは
応　用　編
- 第1章　放射能・放射線事故の歴史
- 第2章　事故のシミュレーションと緊急被ばく医療
- 第3章　汚染や被ばくを伴った患者の診療
- 第4章　局所被ばくの診断と治療
- 第5章　急性放射線症候群の診断と治療
- 第6章　内部被ばくの診断と治療
- 第7章　放射線，核による災害医療

基　礎　編
- 第1章　放射線の人体影響とその機構
- 第2章　放射線測定
- 第3章　線量評価
  - Ⅰ．物理学的線量評価
  - Ⅱ．生物学的線量評価 ―血球による評価
  - Ⅲ．生物学的線量評価 ―染色体異常分析による評価
- 第4章　被ばく医療における放射線管理

資　料　編
- 第1章　原子力災害の体制と法律
- 第2章　わが国の緊急被ばく医療体制

◆ A4判196頁 ◆ 定価（本体 4,700円＋税）
◆ ISBN 978-4-86003-329-3

医療科学社　〒113-0033　東京都文京区本郷 3-23-1　TEL 03-3818-9821　FAX 03-3818-9371
http://www.iryokagaku.co.jp　　（くわしくはホームページをご覧ください）

【改訂新版】あなたと患者のための 放射線防護 Q&A

著者：草間 朋子

知らないことや誤解が多すぎませんか？
患者の疑問や心配に自信をもって答えられますか？
無知や無関心ではすまされない！

知っておきたい医療における放射線防護の必須知識
放射線の影響と被ばくに関する臨床現場からの質問に対し，明快な解答と詳細な解説を付し，さらに防護と管理のあり方を示す。

主要目次

1. 放射線の人体への影響および医療領域における防護の基礎
2. 医療領域で使われる放射線の単位
3. 放射線診療とがんの誘発
4. 放射線診療と白血病
5. 放射線診療と遺伝的影響
6. 低線量放射線被ばくに伴う健康影響
7. 妊娠と放射線診療
8. 放射線診療と不妊
9. 放射線診療と皮膚障害
10. インターベンショナルラジオロジーと患者の防護
11. CTと患者の防護
12. 核医学検査と患者の防護
13. 放射線治療患者の防護
14. 放射線診療従事者自身の防護
15. 女性の放射線診療従事者の防護
16. 知っておく必要のある放射線防護関連法令
17. 放射線影響・防護の視点から見た小児の特徴

◆ A5判160頁　◆ 定価(本体 2,500円＋税)
◆ ISBN 978-4-86003-338-5

医事法セミナー（新版）

著者：前田 和彦

「医療・福祉，社会保障の変化は社会とともにある以上，常に生きた法のあり方を探ることが医事法学である」との著者の理念に基づいた，医療・福祉従事者や一般の読者のための医事法入門書。最新の法改正ならびにその経緯を取り込んで，法の現在をアクチュアルに再生し，装いを改めて刊行！

主要目次

第1講　医事法学とは何か
第2講　医療法
第3講　医療従事者の資格法
第4講　「感染症予防法」と予防衛生法規
第5講　医療契約
　　　　―医療従事者と患者の権利関係―
第6講　医療過誤
第7講　インフォームド・コンセントと患者の自己決定権
第8講　「精神保健福祉法」と保健衛生法規
第9講　社会保障制度の現状
第10講　社会福祉関係法規
第11講　環境衛生法規

◆ A5判224頁　◆ 定価(本体 2,000円＋税)
◆ ISBN 978-4-86003-327-9

医療科学社　〒113-0033 東京都文京区本郷 3-23-1　TEL 03-3818-9821　FAX 03-3818-9371
http://www.iryokagaku.co.jp　（くわしくはホームページをご覧ください）

【医療科学新書】

いずれも 定価（本体1,200円＋税）

リスクマネジメント
医療内外の提言と
放射線部の実践

著者：村上 陽一郎・他
● ISBN978-4-86003-309-5

安全な医療を求める試みは医療界だけの取り組みで達成されるものではない。そこには多角的、学際的な視点が要求されるであろうし、一般から個別を指向する確乎とした哲学が望まれている。本書は、リスクマネジメントの哲学と基礎を提示するとともに、放射線部の個別の試みが一般に敷衍されている実践例を示す。

医療過誤
そのパラダイム

著者：池本 卯典
● ISBN978-4-86003-501-3

著者が、かつて法医学、人類遺伝学、警察の法医鑑識業務などに携りながら体験した、医療過誤にかかわる基礎的問題を整理。医療過誤の頻発を食い止めるためには何をなすべきか、新たなオルタナティブを求めるための思考の枠組みを提示するとともに、医療過誤について問い、答える、学問研究のモデルをも与えてくれる。

医療に活かす癒し術
コ・メディカルのための
医療心理入門

著者：芦原　睦／佐田 彰見
● ISBN978-4-86003-502-0

「現在、医療においては、臓器主義に偏るのではなく、全人的な医療の重要性や、医療心理学の必要性が声高に叫ばれています。その中核に位置するのが、心療内科と考えています」という著者らの臨床（心身医療）と研究に携わった経験をもとに、医療心理学や心身医学を実践していくうえで求められる知識の集成。

日本の疫学
放射線の健康影響研究の
歴史と教訓

著者：重松 逸造
● ISBN978-4-86003-503-7

原爆後障害研究とチェルノブイリ原発事故に果たした疫学の役割と課題。
いまや〈病気の予防と健康に必要な情報を提供する学問〉として広く利用される疫学研究。その指導的役割を戦後半世紀以上にわたって担い、被爆者追跡調査により日本の疫学水準を国際レベルにまで高めた研究の歩みを総括。

放射線物語
！と？の狭間

著者：衣笠 達也
● ISBN978-4-900770-88-1

東海村臨界事故の被曝医療に自らも参加した著者は、放射線の発見から原子力エネルギーの利用に至る歴史、放射線防護の考え方などを平易な言葉で解説しながらも、東海村臨界事故の遠因が、わが国の原子力開発がアメリカからの工学的技術導入に偏り、保健部門の整備が伴っていなかったことにあることを鋭く指摘する。

医療科学社　〒113-0033 東京都文京区本郷 3-23-1　TEL 03-3818-9821　FAX 03-3818-9371
http://www.iryokagaku.co.jp　　（くわしくはホームページをご覧ください）